A M A Z I N G

*in the **second** half*

AMAZING

*in the **second** half*

*Bite sized portions
of wisdom for health,
Happiness and anti-aging
for the over forty crowd.*

Jan Rodenfels

AMAZING in the **Second** Half

ISBN 978-0692665053
Printed in the United States of America

For my husband, Charlie:
You are my best friend, my love,
and my life.
My daughters, Courtney and Alexandra:
You are my heart and my joy.
I am blessed!

CONTENTS

EAT

MOVE

NOURISH

Introduction

This book is for those of us over 40, living life in the "second half." For many, the second half seems a bit scary. We live in a culture that worships youth and we aren't young anymore! Some of us feel that from here on out, everything is downhill. Already suffering from some aches and pains, we wonder if it will get worse. We feel defeated at times when we look in the mirror. Wrinkles are starting to form or are everywhere! Every once in a while we see the face of a friend and find ourselves thinking they suddenly look old. Where did time go and how did all those wrinkles appear?

We also recognize at this time the brevity of life. We begin to go to the funerals of our friends' parents and some of us are now going to the funerals of our friends. Thoughts of our mortality come with each milestone birthday and sometimes with every birthday! There is a fear of dying. A fear experienced by most but often left unspoken. Trust me, everyone thinks about their mortality at least by the time they are 50 years of age.

As a health coach, I believe the second half can be a very exciting time. I know I am excited about this time, though sometimes I find myself calculating how many "good" years I have left. And I knew I wasn't the only one doing this when my friend Doris, wearing her gorgeous, orange Jimmy Choo heels said, "I'm 60 years old and I figure I may have 10 years tops wearing shoes like this!"

The internet and bookshelves are full of 20- and 30-somethings helping us become better versions of ourselves, but they aren't — OK, I'm going to say it — "middle-aged." I am not 30 years old writing this; I am living through middle age myself. Because I am a health coach, people are constantly asking me what I am doing to stay healthy, trim and happy. Some assume, wrongly, that I am starving myself. The exact opposite is true! I love to eat and I eat plenty. I have had to make adjustments with age to keep the healthy body I want, but for me it is an adventure! Finding happiness is about so much more than being thin, although you wouldn't guess that observing our culture. Fulfillment at any age and especially in the second half is only possible with healthy minds, healthy bodies and healthy spirits.

What I want to share with you is a roadmap to living a richer life, one more joyful, more exciting and just as juicy as it was in the first half! I want you to be able to wake up every morning looking forward to the day. You deserve to feel better with each passing day. Even in the second half, life can be an adventure! What fun will old age be if we aren't amazing? We can delay many of the problems of mental and physical aging through self care, a new mindset and work.

If we want our life to be something special in the second half, we need to make some changes. Changes to our thinking, changes to our diets, changes to how we move our bodies, and changes to our very lives. Forget your ancient perceptions of what being older is all about. We all have pasts we may either regret or celebrate, but every day is a new day to be better to ourselves and better to others. Now is the time to learn how we can be the very best versions of ourselves as we go through the second half of life. That is, the Amazing Second Half!

As a certified health counselor, I have coached many second-halfers. Many of them have come to me very frustrated with their weight gain, stressful lives, sleepless nights and lack of energy. They are looking for someone to help them get on the right track. I have often heard, "Just tell me what to eat" or "Tell me what to do." They are sick and tired of being sick and tired, and I don't blame them! We receive conflicting information as well as an overload of information about what to do to achieve optimal health. My job is to help my clients focus on the most important things they can do to get well. I break everything down into bite-sized chunks that people can do to make the necessary changes. I love seeing people get healthy. For me, it is a real joy. This book contains many ways to achieve optimum wellness. It is by no means complete. If it were, it would be a tome. What it is, is the little pearls of wisdom you must know for living the life you want as you grow older — the things that are the essentials. Some of the ideas presented are not new, and others may make you a bit uncomfortable. These, however, are things that need to be said, that our doctors either don't have the time to say or don't know how to say.

I explain to my clients that I am a coach. I cannot do the work for them any more than their basketball or soccer coaches practiced or conditioned for them. A coach is there to guide you, make you better and kick your butt when it needs kicking. A coach can inspire you to be the best version of yourself, but you are the one who must do the hard work. I have witnessed lives transformed when my clients engaged in making positive changes. One diabetic client became a marathon runner and substantially reduced her blood sugar levels that wouldn't budge for years when she changed her diet and added exercise. Another client was able to stop binge eating and lose weight once he discovered his reasons for eating were related to a traumatic childhood event. Although these two clients had completely different situations, they both were ready for change and very coachable.

If you are open to making some changes, you will feel better, look better, sleep better, become more optimistic, lose weight, reduce pharmaceutical use and have less stress. I will share with you my secrets for weight loss, digestive health, stress management, battling sleepless nights and many other things we encounter in the second half of life. You can be AMAZING in the second half! That means looking better, feeling better and having a whole lot more fun!

What's Good About Life in the Second Half?

There are a lot of things that are good in the second half. The first half of our lives we tend to live in our ego. There is so much to prove. We have to make our mark in the world. We collect possessions as if those with the most toys are going to win a prize. We begin as the center of our universe and then, for many of us, our children become the center of the universe. In the second half, we can be humans being, not so much, humans doing. We can be more reflective and take the time to evaluate where it is we want to go and with purpose. For many of us, we are empty nesters. Being alone with our partner can be an awesome time to enjoy each other, to reconnect in a meaningful way, perhaps even to rekindle the romance that brought us together in the first place. Some of us will have grandchildren and great-grandchildren we can enjoy in a way we couldn't before because the demands of career and the bustle of life didn't allow it. The second half is the time to do things we've always wanted to do. The world is our oyster! We can travel, go back to school, start a new career or simply learn something new for the fun of it! Did you know many colleges, universities and community colleges offer tuition waivers for senior citizens? Going back to school may be a wonderful way to explore the subjects you didn't have time for in college. Or, if you never went to college, you can have that experience now!

Some empty nesters are choosing to downsize their living quarters and their possessions in a significant way. In the '60s or '70s, people would stay in their homes or go to retirement communities. Now, they are giving up multi-bedroom houses and taxes, leaving the burbs, moving to the city and relieving themselves of the burden of too many possessions. This new way of life offers freedom and convenience along with the time to do the things people have always wanted to do.

This period in our lives can be a new opportunity to take better care of ourselves — to exercise, to eat better, to take charge of our health. The physiological changes we thought were inevitable with aging are now known to be the result of deconditioning, not age. That is great news!

The second half is also an opportunity to discover who God really is. A God that is greater than we had ever dared in all our "busyness" to hope. It is a time to know God in a much more intimate way.

What's Not So Good in the Second Half?

The second half may not look too good to us if we have let ourselves go — if we haven't exercised, eaten properly, or taken care of ourselves. If we are not at a healthy weight, we will not be at our best. We may be low in energy and even apathetic. If we are not open to trying new things, new adventures, we will stay stuck and miserable in our old age.

Even if we have taken care of ourselves, we live in a culture that doesn't value those of us with experience and wisdom. Our society places a high value on beauty and youth. Psychologist Erik Erickson also suggests that the Western fear of aging keeps us from living full lives. So how can we change that? Every 8 seconds, a baby boomer turns 50, and by 2020 the U.S. population over 65 will have nearly tripled. This demographic represents more than half of the nation's wealth. Marketers are finally realizing that baby boomers present countless profit making opportunities. But how will we see ourselves?

In Japan and China, old age has a much higher status and is associated with wisdom. In Greece, being called an "old man" isn't an insult. The cultural stigma around aging and death does not exist in Greece. In both Greek and Greek-American culture, old age is valued and celebrated. Respect for elders is expected and part of family life.

Today, our longevity is the result of the social progress made throughout history. In a society with so many people over 65, this is a chance for the elderly to be fully participatory in society, especially with our wealth. We can be productive citizens and should occupy a position that contributes to the good of society. We should look to a future of intergenerational fellowship and cooperation. So, how do we change the current atmosphere? Hopefully, our sheer numbers may do that. If this doesn't happen (and it very well may not if our health challenges become a burden on society), the good news is we have each other. There is power in our numbers. We can look to each other for support. The key will be changing the way we perceive ourselves. We must accept beauty in all of the stages of life. We can write about it, talk about it, paint it and live it. Having a sense of humor is also a must. We're surely going to need to laugh a lot!

In addition to taking care of each other, what we must do is take care of ourselves. We live in the land of plenty, we overeat, we move too little. We must become the very best versions of ourselves that we can be. Every step forward on the continuum of health, be it physical, mental or spiritual, will enable us to be productive participants in society as we age and will increase our value. We must not become a burden to our spouses, children, grandchildren or our community at large. There are many things in our lives we cannot control, but making the best choices with regard to our health is something we can and should actively participate in.

Most of us are not living out on a ranch somewhere, going to church on Sundays and looking forward to the monthly dance at the party barn. We are a people on the go with many opportunities to go out to dinner, parties and events. When I have a client that tells me she overindulged at her friend's 50th birthday celebration, I remind her that there will always be another birthday party, just as there will always be the holidays. When we continually "let ourselves go" through all the celebrations of life, we then feel compelled to start the diet roller coaster all over again. Wouldn't it just be easier to enjoy smaller and more nutrient-dense amounts of the things we love and not have to keep starting over? Wouldn't it be better to continually feel good about ourselves?

New Beginnings

"I don't care how old I live;
I just want to be LIVING while I am living!"
-Jack LaLanne

The great thing is that it is never too late to make healthier choices. You can still amaze even yourself! Living in the second half can be your time to start something new. Trying something new is what adds the juiciness to being older. Maybe you are beginning to think about retiring in a few years. Perhaps you have already retired, and you love the time you have to pursue other interests. For some of us, we start a whole new career. I was 50 years old when I launched my second career as a health coach. For me, it was a very exciting time. I loved learning about health, healing and fitness. For years I was like a sponge learning all that I could. People started asking me for advice so I went back to school to build on that hobby, and I was ready to help others with what I knew. Now, I coach executives, handle corporate wellness and do public speaking about health. Many people in the second half are launching new careers that spring forth from their passions. You might want to volunteer more, garden more, paint more, golf more or travel more. Whatever it is you want to do, it is never too late. It is the new beginnings that keep us young — young in spirit, young in our minds. You can enjoy life in the second half.

Skipper and Ezra contacted me six months before Ezra was to retire. Ezra, a top level executive with a major retailer, wanted to get in the best health possible before he retired. Skipper was a successful business coach and wanted to improve her health alongside her husband. They both exercised, but Ezra had always suffered from GI pain and discomfort. Skipper had a few pounds she wanted to lose. They are an amazing couple. They worked on everything I suggested and were open to change. The changes I asked of them were cooking more at home, giving up processed foods, incorporating nutrient dense foods such as leafy greens and eliminating dairy. I upgraded their diets with healthy recipes and they integrated them into their menus. Change is hard for many people but they made no excuses. They just wanted to be the best they could be. Ezra gave up dairy and found relief that he hadn't had in years. Through our sessions,

Ezra and Skipper learned healthier ways to eat, a simpler way to do so, and new techniques for relaxation and stress relief. They recently moved to sunny Florida, drawn to milder winters and a fresh new beginning. They are living their juicy second half!

$$\boxed{\textbf{EAT}}$$

Eat Real Food

"Eat Food. Not too much. Mostly plants."
-Michael Pollan

Food is one of my favorite subjects. Almost all of us love to eat. Food is medicine. We speak to our DNA with every bite we put in our mouths. We may have a predisposition to diabetes or obesity, but every day we have the power to transform that gene expression and reverse disease by changing the messages sent to our DNA. Unfortunately, food is a huge downfall for my clients and most Americans. We eat out too much, our portions are totally out of control and we've gotten away from eating real food. The way we eat has changed more in the last 50 years than it probably had in the 50,000 years before that. Many of the foods we eat are processed. We have evolved to love convenience. The problem with this is that it has ruined our health. Not only is much of our food processed, but it is also full of sugar. Our great grandparents didn't eat this way, nor did their parents. Michael Pollan's quote above, repeated many times, couldn't be said any better! We really are much healthier eating this way, and take it from one who enjoys great tasting food: it doesn't have to be boring, just different.

Maybe it's because I'm a health coach, but people are continually saying to me, "Everything in Moderation." The problem with this statement is that we don't really know what moderation is. Every time I hear this mantra, I see myself channeling Jack Nicholson's character in the movie "A Few Good Men," screaming, "You can't handle the truth!" only I'm shouting, "YOU DON'T KNOW WHAT MODERATION IS!" I do visualize this. Of course, I would never yell that at anyone, but it is my job to help clients find life balance. As a society, we need to find real moderation with regard to our eating, drinking and, for some, our work.

Despite being a health coach, I am not perfect, and I don't expect anyone else to be either. I pretty much follow the 80/20 rule. This rule means I'm 80 percent good with my eating and the other 20 percent I relax and enjoy. When I'm good, I'm making healthy choices and when bad, I'm just a little bit naughty. So if I'm out with friends or family, and they are eating poorly, I am assuming this is their little bit naughty. I am not the food police! Although my daughters and husband would probably say I am the food police, sunscreen officer and security general here at home!

Eat More Plants

If you only take two things from this book, "Eat more plants" would be one of them. Plants are healing, and they are medicine. We do not eat enough plants. Period! I'll say it again; we do not eat enough plants! Americans are good at eating corn, tomatoes, potatoes, lettuce, beans and a few other plants, but there is a whole plethora of vegetables out there we don't seem to appreciate. What we need to do is to eat all the colors of the rainbow, especially dark greens. The brighter the color, the better it is for us. We need about nine servings of fruits and veggies every day. Most of us don't even come close to this. Research has shown us that fruits and vegetables help reduce the risk of heart disease, Type 2 diabetes, some cancers and high blood pressure. Also, it just so happens that if you want to fit into those skinny jeans, fruits and vegetables are what you need a whole LOT more of!

Let's face it: plants aren't the most convenient, which is why many people don't go for them. Eating plants takes a bit of planning and preparation. Not only that, but many of my clients have told me they don't like vegetables. They have bad memories of being told by well-intentioned parents to "eat your vegetables" and even of being forced to finish before getting up from the table.

We need to create a new relationship to plants. I have had to learn to love vegetables myself. I was lucky to have grown up with a family vegetable garden my parents worked hard on. We had lots of corn, beans, and tomatoes, but I don't remember having Chinese cabbage, arugula, bok choy or kale. I had to learn not only to love these veggies but also how to prepare them. I like to think of them as strengthening, beautifying and healing foods! They are all of those things. Plants are also alkaline. We eat many acidic foods that cause our bodies to have a lot of inflammation, and plants heal that inflammation. Generally, acidic foods are meats, fish, grains and alcohol.

I like to think of eating lots of different vegetables as an adventure, a chance to learn something new as I take great care of my body and mind. When I eat vegetables, I visualize the good work they are doing in my body. I also like to find all kinds of amazing ways to prepare them. Learning new ways to cook vegetables makes it exciting. Plus, as we age, any new learning is good for our brains.

Take the time to look at your fruits and vegetables. I mean really look at them. They are completely different in color, texture, shape and size. Every piece of fruit and vegetable has its own personality, its own flavor, its own perfection. There is hardly an end to all the varieties available to us with our global economy. I believe that "seeing" these plants for all that they are, including their beautiful design, is a good step in appreciating all they can do for us.

First Things First

So where do you start to clean up your eating? I say we begin with rising in the morning. This is the place I start with my clients. Breakfast is named breakfast because it means "to break our fast" from the night before. Many people I work with start their day with food or coffee first thing. When we rise, we are dehydrated. The best thing you can do is start with 16 ounces of warm (not hot) purified water. Drink water before you do anything else! Water hydrates us. It makes us feel full so we don't overeat, and it flushes out impurities in our body. It also gets us "moving," if you know what I mean. Or, as one of my favorite clients says, "It makes me poop!" Isn't that what we want? Adding the juice of half an organic lemon to your water is even better. We eat very acidic foods and surprisingly, lemons and limes are alkaline in our bodies, when we might have assumed they were acidic. I always take a full glass of water to the nightstand with me so I can drink it before I get going in the morning. Learning to drink water every morning is an important first step in improving your health.

With age, we don't get the same thirst signals we got when we were young. Understanding this change in our bodies is important. Just because we aren't thirsty doesn't mean we aren't dehydrated.

We can avoid many problems like urinary tract infections, confusion, weakness, pneumonia and even death by staying hydrated. We tend to drink more water if it is flavored. Try adding in organic lemon, lime or cucumbers to water instead of drinking sodas or flavored waters with sugar added. You can fill a pitcher of water at the beginning of the day and make sure it is finished by the end of the day. You can even do this at the office. Once you make a habit of doing this you won't have to think about it; it will be like brushing your teeth.

Our Daily Grind

For many of us, we love our morning ritual that includes coffee. You can just look at the drive-thru at Starbucks every morning to see that. But, what you can also see is the line back at the drive-thru in the afternoon when all that artificial energy has been depleted. Top it all off with some sugar, cream or artificial sweetener, and you have the perfect poison! Some of us can't even imagine our day beginning without coffee. It provides the energy we feel we need to get going in the morning. But coffee is an artificial form of energy. We shouldn't need it to wake up in the morning. If we are eating in a healthy way, exercising and sleeping enough, we should wake up feeling refreshed and ready to go. For most of us, coffee is just a habit, one we are not sure we ever want to give up. To make it harder, the aroma of coffee is so inviting, especially when we have built our little rituals around it.

You might argue that coffee is a plant, a phytonutrient. Yes, you are right about that. There has been a lot of research on the health benefits of coffee. It seems as if there is a new reason to drink coffee every other week! Coffee is big business. We are all bio-individual and some people do well with coffee. In fact, some good research shows that coffee may be protective against some cancers. Other cancers? Not so much. If you are a coffee drinker, you must ask yourself if coffee is helpful to you. I would challenge you to be really honest with yourself. Your health, or lack thereof, depends on it.

You might want to give up your cup of Joe if you have acid reflux, heart palpitations, headaches, ulcers, anxiety, depression, digestive problems or fatigue. If you are overweight, coffee is also harmful to you because it is acidic. Excess acid causes our bodies to produce fat cells so as to keep that acid away from our organs. This is probably not going to help your waistline get any smaller. In fact, high amounts of caffeine make controlling your food cravings and appetite so much harder.

If you realize that coffee is not your friend but need a little more convincing, here are just a few other reasons to give it up. First of all, it stains your pearly whites. Second, your breath smells bad and, last but not least, unless your coffee is organic, your beans have been doused with an unhealthy dose of pesticides. So, it really is poison! In this case, buy organic.

I know I will not be very popular with my take on coffee, but I must be honest with you. People who really love their coffee really love it! I get that! I don't think I would have gotten through calculus or anatomy without it. It really helped me to focus for extended periods of time when I needed it. What I decided concerning coffee was that it would be an occasional treat for me. First, I went cold turkey with no coffee for two months to get rid of the addiction. I had a mild headache for the first three or four days, and then it went away. Symptoms of withdrawal will differ by individual depending on how much caffeine you have consumed. You can wean off even more easily by cutting the coffee (and all caffeinated drinks) in half for the first week or two. This makes for a more gradual withdrawal. Just be sure to keep paring your consumption down! Now, I enjoy one cup of coffee if I go out to breakfast on the weekend, if I'm a guest in someone's home, or if I have guests in my home that drink coffee. I often drink a cup before a race but not while I am training. This way I don't feel deprived. I can still enjoy it a bit, but caffeine doesn't own me anymore. Try it! See how much better you feel and how much weight you lose.

If you need to replace your cup of Joe, try herbal teas like chamomile, peppermint, lemon balm, passionflower, rosemary, sage, and thyme. There is also chaga, a fungus that comes off of a tree and is then pounded out to make tea. Many of these teas offer the benefits of antioxidants, anti-inflammatory and immune-stimulating properties. There is even some preliminary research that suggests that chaga may be good for fighting inflammatory bowel disease and diabetes and for inhibiting cancer cell growth (although currently there is a lack of clinical trial research). The addition of these teas nourishes you with phytonutrients, vitamins and minerals. Plus, they provide something warm to drink and help create a new morning ritual.

Last year, Bill turned 59 and was feeling really lousy and not on top of his game. He had gained back 40 of the 70 pounds he had worked so hard to lose many years ago. Bill was drinking 6 to 8 cups of caffeinated coffee each day. Having spent years chasing all of the newest fad diets, he said he didn't want to "feel shitty" when he hit 60. It was a big change for him to give up sugar, dairy, most gluten, and his beloved coffee. The first week was awful, with headaches and sleepiness. Now, he reports that he sleeps better, has increased energy and has lost substantial weight. He is down 30 pounds at this writing. His cholesterol is ridiculously low, and he says he doesn't miss coffee at all now. Bill has replaced his coffee with chaga. In fact, it was Bill who shared chaga with me. I love learning new ways to improve health!

Breakfast

Breakfast is the most important meal of the day. I feel very strongly about this because I have seen it work not only for my clients but for myself. It is the meal that sets the pace for the whole day.

One of my first clients was morbidly obese and lost 17 pounds just by eating breakfast. He hadn't changed anything else at that point. He is a very busy executive who just didn't believe he had time to eat, and he thought skipping breakfast would help him lose weight. Not so! After beginning a breakfast routine, what he found was he had more time because he could concentrate better. He also felt better thanks to the weight loss. He said he hadn't realized how bad he had felt. Eating breakfast had actually jump-started his sluggish metabolism.

Many Americans eat cereal for breakfast. It's easy, and it tastes good to most people. But it is junk food. Breakfast cereal is processed and usually loaded with sugar. It is made by taking grains in their whole, nutritious state and moving them to a highly processed, nutritionally depleted state. Many of my clients do not like hearing this. I totally understand because I grew up on cereal as most of us baby boomers did. I also grew up on Pop-Tarts and Carnation Instant Breakfast. Holy Cow! When I was in high school, this was my go-to breakfast most school days (I was a real sugar addict then). It is a known fact that the more our food is processed, the more natural nutrients are lost. When we were young, we could probably get away with eating a bad breakfast, although I'm not at all sure I got away with a thing. My sugary breakfast probably accounts for the fact that I was always the last one chosen for any sport at school! But that's a story for another time.

So, what should we eat for breakfast? Well, we are all bio-individual. What works for me isn't necessarily what is going to work for you. That being said, make sure you know what's right for you. If your weight isn't where it should be, examine your current choices. Try new breakfasts. I suggest you not think of the typical American breakfast. Think outside the box. It could be steel cut oats with berries, a smoothie or leftovers from dinner. Many cultures eat much differently for breakfast than we do. They might have rice, fish or even lamb for the first meal of the day.

Eat eggs but not bacon. Bacon is processed and increases the risk of cancer (as do sausage and hot dogs). Bacon is also high in fat, cholesterol, and sodium. It can increase your risk of diabetes, heart disease, and various types of cancer. According to the American Institute of Cancer Research (AICR), just 1.7 ounces of processed meats consumed daily can increase a person's risk for colorectal cancer by 21 percent. That is less than two slices of bacon a day. The AICR found that regular intake of even small amounts of cold cuts and bacon increased the risk of cancer and so recommends avoiding these foods.

I know for many, bacon tastes great, and many dishes contain bacon. Who doesn't love a BLT? I sure do! Does this mean I NEVER eat bacon? No, but I don't eat bacon or processed foods at home, and when I eat out and it's on a salad I ask them to leave it off. Occasionally, when I go to my favorite weekend breakfast spot, Fox in the Snow, I let owner Lauren leave it on the best egg sandwich in town (it's a small piece of bacon!). This tiny piece of bacon is my little indulgence, and it's OK. I don't worry when I am eating healthy most of the time. And in full disclosure, I have it with her made-from-scratch pecan roll. Amazing!

Eggs are not the bad food we were told in the past. If you have no allergy to them, they can be a fine choice. In fact, eggs have many nutrients and are a good protein in a vegetarian diet. They are very satisfying, particularly the yolk. I don't recommend eating just egg whites. Eat the creamy yellow center; that's where the nutrition lies. We need some fat to regulate our hormones. When we cut out fat, we start to have out-of-control cravings. Choose organic, free-range eggs as they are better for us and the planet. Learn to eat eggs with greens like baby kale, baby spinach or arugula. Sauté onions, mushrooms, tomatoes or any veggie you love to jazz them up.

Toast, cereal, muffins and donuts are not our friends. I recommend eating a simple, clean breakfast of gluten-free steel cut oats and organic berries. Back in the day, I cooked steel cut oats for 45 to 50 minutes. I just hated making them because they took so long! Because they did, I only made them on the weekends. Now, I use the Arrowhead Mills brand of gluten-free steel cut oats because I can cook them in 12 minutes, which is quick enough for me even on busy days. I choose organic berries because they are so healthy for us, and they are the best fruit to keep from elevating our blood sugar levels. I buy fresh in season and frozen out of season. If you are overweight or diabetic, berries are your ideal fruit choice. If you are at your ideal weight and not eating a lot of sweets, other fruits that are in season are perfectly good choices and they all have their own individual benefits. I recommend staying with berries if you still have weight to lose or are diabetic.

Brown rice is a wonderful breakfast food and is very nourishing. I soak the grains in water overnight or all day before cooking. Many people do not know that soaking grains and legumes is important. Grains contain phytic acid which interferes with the absorption of zinc, calcium, iron and other essential minerals. All that is needed is to cover them with water in a bowl and then strain off the water before cooking. In Paul Pitchford's book "Healing With Whole Foods," he discusses the fact that whole brown rice is concentrated in B vitamins and beneficial for the nervous system. When cooking brown rice for dinner, I make extra in my rice cooker to have it for breakfast the next day. I love it with toasted pumpkin seeds and umeboshi plum on top (see recipe on page 142). It tastes amazing!

Concerning breakfast, you are only limited by your imagination. You might make extra fish the night before and eat with vegetables or a small amount of brown rice. Like I said before, you don't need to eat the typical American breakfast. It's much better for you if you don't!

I will tell you what I eat 90 percent of the time. I have my water, I often juice veggies in the juicer, go workout or shower, and then I have a smoothie or steel cut oats. How many grains I have depends on how much physical activity I am doing. If I'm going for a long run, I need something like oatmeal. If I'm having a very unusual day and will not be working out at all, I have no grains, just a protein like eggs and veggies, or a smoothie with fruit and a raw vegan protein powder. This is one of the ways I control my weight.

I do love smoothies. This is a great way to sneak a green vegetable in like kale, spinach, parsley or microgreens with berries. You'll hardly even know it's there, and when you are done, you will have consumed two of your body's daily requirement of fruits and vegetables. I add in some superfoods to my smoothie, like maca, goji berries, raw cacao, and chia seeds (see Building a Smoothie on page 24). Sometimes I alternate the superfoods, and sometimes I add them all in a single smoothie. It just depends how much I am exercising and where my weight is. The base of my smoothies is either cashew or almond milk. Coconut milk is fine too. There is no right or wrong way to make a smoothie; it is up to your personal taste. Some of my clients like their smoothies watery, and some like it a bit thick as I do — thick enough to eat with a spoon. This gives me the satisfaction of eating a meal. Whichever way you like to drink a smoothie, it is important to chew your drink. Why chew a drink? Because digestion begins in the mouth and your saliva will mix with the ingredients to aid in digestion.

Need more convincing that breakfast is a good idea? One brand new study reveals that skipping breakfast makes you more likely to suffer a stroke. This 15-year study carried out in Osaka, Japan, of 130,000 men and women aged 45 and older found that the more days a week participants had breakfast, the lower their risk of suffering a stroke. Not only that, but another large study, 16 years in the making, found that men who skipped breakfast had a 27 percent higher risk of heart attack or death from coronary heart disease than those who started the day with something in their bellies. This study even accounted for differences in diet, exercise and smoking as it tracked 26,902 male health professionals, ages 45 to 82. All of the men were second-halfers! This study did not include women, but I think we may assume similar outcomes.

Building A Smoothie

Choose one or two items from each category and create your own drink!

When I teach a class on making smoothies, I always say, "It's a smoothie, not rocket science!" Even so, the pros usually start with hard, chunky ingredients like frozen fruits, nuts and seeds so they go close to the blades. Next are soft, chunky ingredients like greens, fresh fruit, nut butters, tofu, etc. Third are the powders and superfood add-ins. Then comes the liquid and, lastly, ice. Some people really like ice in a smoothie. I prefer no ice, especially if I'm using frozen fruit in winter. It is already cold enough!

Base	Liquid (1-2 cups)	Cream
Fruits, Fresh Fruits, Frozen Carrot Cucumber	Coconut Water Water Green Tea Almond Milk Coconut Milk	Avocado Banana Mango Silken Tofu Nut Butter (1-2 T) Raw Nuts (1/4 cup)

Greens (1-2 cups)	Super Food Add-Ins (1/2-1 T)	Tasty Add-Ins (as you like)

Alfalfa
Chard
Kale
Romaine
Spinach
Beet Greens
Collard Greens
Mustard Greens
Cilantro
Mint
Parsley
	Chia Seeds
	Goji Berries
	Ground Flax
	Maca
	Spirulina (1/4 tsp)
	Dulse Flakes
	Protein Power
	(1 scoop)
	Coconut Oil
	Hemp
	Flax Oil
	Olive Oil
	Raw Nuts or Seeds
	Raw Cacao
		Sweetener:
		  Dates
		  Stevia
		  Maple Syrup
		  Agave
		  Brown Rice Syrup
		Spices:
		  Cinnamon
		  Tumeric
		  Ginger
		  Nutmeg
		  Chai spices
		Zest:
		  Lemon
		  Lime
		Natural Extracts:
		  Vanilla
		  Almond
		  Peppermint
		Herbs:
		  Mint
		  Basil
		  Parsley
		  Cilantro

Snack Attack

Having a snack mid-morning and then again after lunch helps keep our blood sugar balanced and prevents overeating when we sit down to a meal. What we eat when snacking is crucial for good health. Get rid of those sugary and processed snacks and make much better choices. Snack choice is a key to looking and feeling amazing!

One of the best snacks is nuts. Nuts have been proven to help people lose weight and reduce the risk of diabetes. They are great because they are chock full of protein, minerals, fiber and healthy fats. Choose only nuts that are raw or lightly toasted without salt. The best to choose from are almonds, walnuts, pecans, macadamia, and hazelnuts. Be careful to eat only a small amount as too many can raise your blood sugar. A ¼ cup is best or about 10 to 12 nuts. Always premeasure and place in small snack bags, so you are not tempted to overeat.

Brazil nuts are full of selenium, in fact, more than any other food. Selenium is known for producing antioxidants, regulating thyroid hormone and supporting the immune system. However, too much selenium can lead to selenium toxicity or selenosis. Signs of selenosis include hair loss, skin rashes, nausea, fatigue and mood changes. If you like Brazil nuts, eat just one or two of them to reap the benefits without any worries. In fact, a Harvard study of selenium shows that men with higher levels of selenium had a 48 percent reduced risk of prostate cancer than those with the lowest levels. More than half of U.S. men have less than ideal levels of selenium. Take two Brazil nuts a day and you may just keep prostate cancer away!

Planning your snacks in advance can keep you on track and eating right. Prep your favorite raw veggies by washing and chopping them so they are ready to go when you want them. Most of us reach for unhealthy snacks because of convenience. For making good choices, convenience is everything. Buy or make hummus for a dip if you like. If buying hummus, take your reading glasses and make sure the only oil in the ingredient list is olive. Many brands use the undesirable oils. Another good choice for a snack is an apple with almond or peanut butter. Be sure to measure the nut butter. One tablespoon is plenty.

Superfoods

Although there is no legal or medical definition of a superfood, superfoods are nutritional powerhouses that pack large doses of vitamins, minerals, antioxidants and polyphenols. Eating superfoods is believed to reduce the risk of chronic disease and cancer and to prolong life. Superfoods are mostly plants, but some fish and dairy also qualify. Below is a list of my favorite superfoods that you can integrate into a healthy diet.

1. Flax and Chia Seeds

Over the course of human evolution, we have made a dramatic change in the ratio of omega-6 to omega-3 fats that we consume. It may be this change as much as any other dietary factor that has contributed to our epidemic of modern disease. Our hunter-gatherer ancestors were probably consuming omega-6 to omega-3 fats in a ratio of about 1-to-1. Today, estimates of that ratio range from an average of 20-to-1, with some individuals as high as 25-to-1. Both chia and flax seeds are high in omega-3s.

Chia seeds hold 30 times their weight in water and are chock full of fiber. They also keep you feeling full for a long time and, therefore, are very helpful for weight loss. I eat a tablespoon every day in my smoothie, on my oatmeal or in salads.

Flax seeds are ranked as the number one source of lignans in human diets. Lignans are unique fiber-related polyphenols that provide antioxidant benefits for anti-aging, hormone balance and cellular health. They also support the growth of probiotics in the gut. Using flax regularly may help reduce the number or severity of colds and flu. They protect the digestive tract and maintain GI health. Flax seeds are beneficial for those suffering from Crohn's disease. Be sure to grind your flax seeds in a nut or coffee grinder right before use. Use 1 to 2 tablespoons per day.

2. Blueberries

You have to love this cute little North American fruit because it packs a powerful nutritional punch. Blueberries are an antioxidant superfood. Blueberries are packed with antioxidants and phyto-flavinoids and are high in potassium and vitamin C. Not only can they lower your risk of heart disease and cancer, but their anti-inflammatory properties ease pain and slow disease. Plus, they fight wrinkles! These little berries are a perfect fruit for diabetics. Ideally, you should try for ½ to 1 cup a day. Buy organic, frozen or fresh.

3. Wild Salmon

Salmon is full of omega-3 fatty acids, protein, potassium, selenium, B vitamins, and vitamin D. One study found that women who ate omega-3-rich fish twice a week significantly lowered their risk of heart failure later in life. Another study found that eating just 3 ounces of salmon twice per week can increase levels of HDL (the good cholesterol), compounds essential in maintaining a healthy circulatory system. Salmon has also been found to provide protection from UV-induced skin damage. And for us middle-agers, the DHA in salmon has been linked to improved cognitive function. Eat twice a week and only 3 ounces per serving, being sure to buy wild salmon.

4. Walnuts

Chock full of protein, fiber, vitamins, minerals and more omega-3s: Is there anything left to say? Eating just a handful a day will help lower cholesterol, boost brain power, reduce the effects of stress, fight cancer, promote sleep and prevent heart disease. A new study shows that walnuts appeared to lower the risk of breast cancer in mice. Eat five (1-ounce) servings a week. Nuts make a great snack!

5. Avocados

Avocados may be high in fat, but it's the heart-healthy kind — monounsaturated fatty acids. These delicious fruits also include 20 different vitamins and minerals. How's that for a superfood? A single 3.5-ounce serving has only 9 grams of carbs, 7 of which are fiber, so you actually "net" 2 carbs, making this a perfect low-carb plant food. Avocados have more potassium than bananas. Potassium matters because studies have shown that a high potassium intake is linked to reduced blood pressure, a major risk factor for stroke, heart attack and kidney failure. The oleic acid in avocados has been associated with reduced inflammation. The heart-healthy fat in avocados helps you absorb the nutrients in plant foods. Some nutrients are "fat soluble," meaning that they need to be combined with fat for our bodies to utilize that good stuff! Avocados are also good for the eyes and may help prevent cancer. They taste rich and creamy too!

6. Goji Berries

Most of us did not grow up eating goji berries, known as the "longevity fruit." These berries are native to Tibet and Inner Mongolia and have been used by Chinese herbalists for centuries to treat visual ailments and poor circulation and to boost the immune system. While these claims may not be supported by scientific research yet, there is no denying that goji berries are rich in antioxidants, full of vitamins A and C, iron and calcium. The goji berry is an "adaptogen," a term used to describe plants that increase the body's resistance to stress. Adaptogens survive in harsh climates, and because they have adapted to these harsh conditions, they have highly concentrated nutrients that are believed to help our bodies cope with stress, provide energy and maintain an active immune system. Put them in your smoothie or eat them right out of the bag. I like the Navitas Naturals brand. Eat 1 ounce (100 calorie snack!).

7. Kale

Kale packs in more nutrition than almost any other food. One cup of chopped kale has 2.4 grams of fiber, 100 milligrams of calcium, and 239 milligrams of potassium — that's 14 percent of your daily calcium, 659 percent of vitamin A and more than 900 percent of your vitamin K! And cooked kale offers more iron per ounce than beef. This vibrant green is nutrient dense, and that's what our bodies need. Just make sure to pair it with a healthy fat (coconut oil, olive oil, avocado), as some of its nutrients are hard for the body to absorb.

8. Romaine Lettuce

That Caesar salad may just be better than you think! Romaine packs high levels of folic acid, a water-soluble form of vitamin B. It's also not quite as bitter as some of the best leafy greens and, therefore, a favorite among many.

9. Parsley

I like to think of parsley as the quiet green. Usually relegated to the side of our plate as a garnish, it is often overlooked. It is a nutritional powerhouse; even one sprig can go a long way towards your daily requirement of vitamin K. Research has also suggested that the aroma and flavor of parsley may help control your appetite. Parsley is also great for improving one's breath. Chew a sprig of this herb, chop it up in a salad or drop some in your blender when making a smoothie.

10. Raw Cacao

If you love chocolate, raw cacao is the best way to get all of its benefits. This Mayan superfood has been consumed for centuries, but I'm not talking about the chocolate you are eating in candy bars. It is nutrient dense chocolate without the sugar and processing. Raw cacao is the bean of the cacao plant that is the source for all chocolate and cocoa products. In its raw form, cacao maintains higher levels of antioxidants, vitamin C, phenethylamine (PEA, the feel-good neurotransmitter responsible for the feeling of love), omega-6 fatty acids, tryptophan, and serotonin. All the bad things associated with non-raw chocolate, like cavities, weight gain and diabetes, are caused by the fillers added to dark chocolate — ingredients such as sugar, milk, and other fillers. This raw chocolate is healthy for you. Cacao is the highest food source of magnesium, which happens to be one of the minerals we, in our modern culture, are the most deficient in. As an antioxidant, raw cacao blows red wine, blueberries and green tea out of the water. It's great for the heart, it's good for diabetics and it' not toxic to the liver. One tablespoon is only 20 calories! Throw in your smoothie in powder form or, better yet, eat raw chocolate nibs.

The White Menace

No, I'm not talking about snow! The "white menace" is probably at the root of all our diseases and the reason so many of us are overweight. The white menace includes refined flour, refined white sugar, white rice and potatoes. In other words, cereals, bagels, cakes, cookies, pasta, bread, ice cream, mac and cheese, and so many of our comfort foods. When I am working with clients, this seems to be one of the toughest areas for people to make changes. As a recovered sugar addict, I totally understand this. Pop-Tarts and Carnation Instant Breakfast used to just call my name! When I could finally give these menacing foods up, amazing things started to happen. My skin cleared up, my energy levels went through the roof and I felt more relaxed. The white menace was not my friend! Trust me; there are much better choices.

I could write about all the latest research on insulin imbalance and "diabesity" from eating the white menace, but there are plenty of books out there that have done this. One of my favorites is Dr. Mark Hyman's book "The Blood Sugar Solution." As a functional medicine doctor, he understands that food is medicine. I use his protocol for my clients with diabetes, and it works very well. What I prefer to do here is motivate you to make changes as if your life depended on it, because it does. And as my clients continually say to me, "Just tell me what to eat!" I have come to realize that many of us are totally confused about what we should be eating. We get many conflicting messages in the media telling us what to eat or not to eat: "Coffee is good for you," "Coffee is bad for you," "Eggs are good," "Eggs are bad," "Fat is bad for you," "Fat is good for you." Someone once said that nutrition is a fledgling science. I believe that is true. One thing I do know is that refined carbohydrates are making us sick. When people give this stuff up, they get well, and they lose weight. This white stuff also makes you tired. Seriously reducing or, ideally, eliminating the white menace may very likely keep you from having a heart attack, cancer, high blood pressure or obesity. You will then sleep better, have more energy and — the bonus is — you will look Amazing!

Concerning sugar, we all need a little sweetness in our lives. I look ahead at the week, and if I am going to an exclusive restaurant or know I will be entertaining and making dessert, I wait and savor my reward for these times. We do not need dessert every day. When we crave something sweet, often our bodies are looking for some fat. You might try avocado or almond butter and see if the craving passes.

Below is the list of foods you should not eat when cutting back on the white menace as well as a list of foods you can eat. Fortunately, the list of things you can eat is much longer than the list of those you shouldn't. Whoo-whoo! For weight loss, it is best to go cold turkey on all the white menace. You can pick one cheat day to have a favorite treat, just not the whole pint of Ben and Jerry's! When you are at your ideal weight, it is fine to have, say, a sandwich on bread occasionally. Picking an organic sprouted grain, whole wheat, or a good gluten-free bread, occasionally, is fine, but your best bet to be amazing is eating real whole grains. Remember, even whole wheat bread is processed. Steel cut oats, brown rice, millet, amaranth and the like are the whole grains I am talking about.

Eating These Foods = Not Amazing

All-Purpose Flour	Bread	Crackers
Cake Flour	Bagels	Tortilla Chips
Pastry Flour	Pastries	Jam
Whole Wheat Flour	Cakes	Jelly
Unbleached Flour	Candy	Teriyaki Sauce
Rice Flour	Cookies	Many Salad Dressings
Brown Rice Flour	Sodas	
Rye Flour	Ice Cream	
Corn Flour	Pasta	

Eating these foods = Amazing

Vegetables and Legumes	Fruits
Avocados	Apples
Lettuce	Berries
Chard	Cherries
Cabbage	Figs
Broccoli	Apricots
Carrots	Melons
Celery	Peaches
Bell peppers	Pears
Cauliflower	Bananas
Squash	Nectarines
Green Beans	Papaya
Tomatoes	Mangoes
Radishes	Pineapple
Bok choy	Dried fruits
Endive	Grapes
Kale	Fruit preserves (no sugar added)
Spinach	
Beans (black, white, kidney, garbanzo)	
Peas (sugar snap peas, snow peas, English peas)	

Starches and Grains

Oats

Amaranth

Millet

Farro

Rice (brown and wild)

Sweet potatoes and yams

Quinoa

Corn and corn meal

Arrowroot powder

Nuts and Seeds

Almonds

Cashews

Peanut butter and other nut butters(no sugar added)

Pecans

Pistachios

Pumpkin seeds

Sesame seeds

Soy nuts

Sunflower seeds

Walnuts

Tahini

Meat, Poultry and Fish*

Chicken

Beef

Turkey

Shellfish

Pork

Eggs

Fish (especially wild salmon and mackerel)

Dairy*

Yogurt (plain)

Milk (organic)

cheese

Sweets

Stevia

Maple syrup(pure)

honey(raw)

* Reducing the amount of animal products or, ideally, eliminating them is one of the best things we can do for our health. There are many studies to back up this statement. I must add that I don't believe dairy is good for us either. We are the only species on the planet that continues to drink milk after infancy and also drinks the milk of another species. With all our dairy consumption, we Americans have very high levels of osteoporosis. I suggest reading further on this subject (see Recommended Reading, page 161). Many people also have an allergy to dairy. Dairy has been forced on us for decades. The dairy industry is a multibillion-dollar industry that has very creative ways to keep us unhealthy and fat, eating cheese, butter, and milk. If you want to continue eating dairy, I would suggest all your dairy products be organic. At least this way, you will not be getting all the antibiotics, pesticides, steroids and hormones found in milk products.

WARNING: Eliminating the white menace will cause weight loss!

Eat Fat, Lose Weight

Eating fat sounds crazy coming from a health coach doesn't it? Eating fat is counterintuitive to what we've been advising for so long. For decades, we've been told by scientists, nutritionists, doctors, and even our government to eat a low-fat, low-carb diet to lose weight. Or, we were told to change up our carbs and eat whole wheat bread and whole wheat pasta. Unfortunately, we are fatter and sicker than ever before following this advice.

The science does not support eating this way now. The idea that a low-fat diet is "healthy" is one of the biggest nutrition lies there ever was! In fact, there is currently better science that confirms we need to eat more fat. There is good reason to be excited about this, but don't run out and order fried chicken and a greasy hamburger! There are good fats and bad fats, but before I get to those, let me tell you about one study that supports this idea.

On the Island of Kitava, one of the Trobriand Islands in the Papua, New Guinea archipelago, the Islanders showed no signs of heart disease or stroke. The results of a study called the Kitava Study are very impressive and particularly interesting for those of us in the second half. The oldest residents had a good quality of life and lived fully up until their deaths. They ate a diet of up to 21% saturated fat from coconuts and had no heart disease. This lack of heart disease was unanimously confirmed by doctors and researchers. In fact, there were no indications of dementia, diabetes, acne, obesity, and no high blood pressure.

These islanders of Kitava lived exclusively on root vegetables (yams, taro, tapioca, sweet potato), fruits including banana, papaya, pineapple, mango, guava, watermelon, and pumpkin, vegetables, fish and coconuts. We would be much healthier if we ate this way. Notice there are no breads, sugar, or processed foods in their diet.

What we need is an oil change! Get rid of trans fats, hydrogenated oils, fried foods and the bad oils like canola, safflower, peanut, and sunflower.

Eliminate refined carbs like bread, and plates of pasta. Together, sugar and carbs are the true cause of weight gain. Eating saturated fat with carbs is deadly, think bread and butter. One of the worst meals you may be making is spaghetti and garlic bread, a classic American favorite!

When we eat omega-3 fats (sometimes called the happy fats), we won't need Prozac. Consuming foods like wild fish, flax and chia seeds, wild game, and whole eggs will provide these omega-3's. Healthy fats will cut your cravings! When we have cravings for dessert and the like, we are in reality looking for fat. Eating good fats helps your body release fat, balance hormones and improve your sex life. Include fats like avocado, nuts, butter (from grass fed cows), and if you choose to eat beef, eat grass fed beef. Coconut oil is one of the healthiest plant-based fats that will keep you satisfied. Coconut oil contains medium-chain triglycerides (MCTs), a saturated fatty acid that has many health benefits, ranging from improved cognitive function to weight loss. MCTs have largely been missing from standard western diets. We now know that MCT oils should be consumed every day. I put coconut oil in my smoothie every morning, and I get smarter and smarter! Enjoy the good fats and bite by bite you can change your body and your health!

Read Food Labels

Reading labels is something you need to do. You have to count on yourself to stay healthy. You must be your best advocate. You can't rely on the government, and you can't rely on the company packaging your food. What you can do is read labels. Every packaged food is required to list the ingredients. If you can't pronounce the word, if you have never heard of it, or if it ends in -ose, don't buy it. If the list includes hydrogenated oils, artificial flavors or preservatives, put that package back on the shelf. You don't want it, and neither does your body. And don't even think of trusting words on the packaging like "natural," "wholesome" or even "nutritious."

Ingredients are listed on a package in descending order by weight, including added water. Remember that the ingredient listed first is present in the largest amount. So the ingredient list is all about quantity, but that doesn't always tell the whole story. For example, a jar of salsa may list tomatoes first, so you know that there are more tomatoes in there than anything else. But when it comes to sugar, sodium, and saturated and trans fats, it's hard to tell how much is in there. All of these ingredients, if in excess, can damage your heart and increase your risk of stroke. It is important to know these ingredients by their aliases. Salt goes by sodium benzoate, sodium nitrite, and monosodium glutamate (MSG), to name a few. Sugar can go by agave nectar, corn syrup, high-fructose corn syrup, barley malt syrup, dehydrated cane juice and other names. Trans fats are even trickier because they aren't mentioned as trans fats in the ingredient list. They are disguised mostly as partially hydrogenated oil and hydrogenated oil. These trans fats can raise your bad cholesterol (LDL) and lower your good cholesterol (HDL). They are also known to elevate your risk of heart disease and stroke. Don't eat this stuff!

You're Sweet Enough

I know I mentioned sugar in the context of the white menace, but I think this needs a bit more attention. We Americans eat a crazy amount of sugar. More than any other country in the world. Did you know that in the 1600s, here in the USA, we consumed on average about 6 to 10 pounds of sugar per year, per person? Sounds like a reasonable amount if you think about a five-pound bag of the white stuff. Now, imagine us today, eating an average of 150 to 185 pounds of refined sugars! That would be about 37 five-pound bags of sugar, per person, in one year! And let's remember, that's the average. Many people are eating much more.

Living in the land of plenty, we have gone completely bonkers on the stuff, and what's more, many of us don't realize how much sugar is hidden in so many of our foods. Processed sugar hides in everything from tomato sauce and salad dressing to crackers and bread. What's more, the snack industry spends over ten billion dollars annually to lure us into eating even more of the stuff.

How sugar works in our bodies is important. Refined sugars enter the bloodstream quickly (we can actually absorb sugar right through our cheeks). It's instant energy. No wonder people are in line for their caramel macchiato! The body then converts these foods to glucose. The glucose triggers our pancreas to secrete insulin to convert the excess glucose into glycogen for storage in our liver and muscles. Any unmetabolized calories are then stored as fat. So we gain weight. You also have excess insulin in your body and some inflammation. Sugar in and of itself does not cause diabetes, but lifestyle is a major risk factor, and sugar is usually accompanied by refined white flour in desserts, breads and cereals. Eating too much of these kinds of foods could lead you to become insulin resistant. Insulin resistance leads to prediabetes or Type 2 diabetes. Excess insulin in the body can harden blood vessels, damage arterial walls and increase cholesterol and blood pressure.

Sugar provides our bodies with empty calories. While we may receive energy from sugar, there are no nutrients. What results is that we eat more without ever feeling satisfied. Overeating leads to a risk of weight gain and to a continuous cycle of highs and lows in our energy levels. Sugar is also correlated with depression; countries with the highest sugar intakes report the highest rates of depression. High sugars have been linked to cancer as well, and for those with cancer, sugar may be fuel for the cancer cells, although further research is needed to understand this connection completely.

So, how much sugar should we eat? If you trust the government (not sure why we would), the USDA reports that we can have up to 10 teaspoons per day. Other sources like the American Heart Association (AHA) suggests the maximum amount of sugar per day for men is 37.5 grams or 9 teaspoons. The amount for women is 25 grams or 6 teaspoons per day. Through experimentation and client reports, I believe the AHA numbers to be the best. We would all do much better to eat less sugar. If we are going to eat less sugar, it is necessary to read nutrition labels. Labels list the amount of sugar in grams. We can convert the grams to teaspoons by dividing the grams by four. For example, if your yogurt label states that it contains 26 grams of sugar, you can quickly convert this quantity into teaspoons: 26 grams divided by 4 equals 6.5 teaspoons of sugar per serving.

For a woman, this one serving of yogurt would represent the recommended daily supply of sugar. Not only are you getting dairy (potentially complete with hormones and antibiotics), but, in one fell swoop, you are getting all the sugar you should have in one day. If you just love yogurt and do not want to give it up, an upgrade would be to buy plain organic yogurt and add fresh or frozen fruit.

Before asking my clients to cut back on sugar, I work at getting them to increase healthy, nutrient-dense foods first. I have found that if they are eating a lot of simple carbs and animal protein, they are not successful in reducing sugar. Adding lots of greens to your diet and reducing animal foods makes it much easier to get rid of this junk.

Cutting back sugar intake takes some real work, but it is very doable with a bit of awareness. Because we are all so bio-individual, what works for one person doesn't work for another. Once we have implemented good clean food, some of us, including myself, prefer going cold turkey with sugar. If I have a little sugar, I continue wanting more. It's as if there is a monster in my belly just waiting to be fed sugar. Once I have gone cold turkey for a week or so, I can allow myself a treat once a week, and I have no problem. If I have sugar two days in a row, I am lured right back on the sugar.

Other people have success weaning off sugar more slowly. Looking at labels and keeping track of how many grams they eat each day brings an awareness that results in self-control. This knowledge of the sugar they are consuming helps to reduce consumption. Whichever path you take to reduce sugar will make a huge difference in your energy levels, weight, and overall health. Don't forget to give yourself a lot of credit and a big pat on the back for making this significant change!

Should I Take Supplements?

Yes, and here's why. Many of us are nutrient malnourished. First, our soils are not what they used to be. There is no longer the amount of minerals that our ancestors enjoyed. We live in an environment that is toxic both in the air we breathe and the water we drink. In addition, we enjoy an abundance of junk food, food that is highly processed and lacking in nutrients. Many of us spend a lot of time indoors, and we have a deficiency of sunlight. We may also have added stress in our lives, and combating this requires much better nutrients than we are probably getting through food sources.

At the very least, everyone needs a good multivitamin, omega-3 fatty acids, and probably a probiotic. When you buy supplements, make sure they are the highest quality you can buy. I wouldn't suggest getting your supplements at a drugstore. I prefer supplements that are high quality, high potency, whole food vitamins and minerals. Good quality supplements will include whole foods you might find in the grocery store, like peas, radishes and beets. Look for these from a trusted health food store. Concerning supplements, remember that more is not necessarily better. Just because a multivitamin offers a large variety of supplements doesn't mean it is better for you. In fact, there are some supplements you don't want to take, which may be in multivitamins (see below). Also, remember that supplements are just that; they are there to boost a healthy diet, to fill in the gaps when we don't get what we need in our food. Listed below are some recommended supplements:

1. A good multivitamin – Find a good whole food brand like Mega Foods. You want to make sure your multivitamin does not have a high dose of isolated vitamin E (200 IU or greater), folic acid (you want folate instead) or copper. You may not want added iron in your multivitamin. Guidance from a health coach or a nutritionally oriented physician can help you pick the one best for you.

2. Vitamin D3 – Vitamin D has been touted as the wonder vitamin for the last several years. We have been told that we need supplementation because most of us are deficient (perhaps as much as 80% of the population). It has been said that vitamin D offers protection against some cancers, osteoporosis, heart attack, Alzheimer's and other chronic conditions. Vitamin D improves metabolism by influencing more than 200 different genes. You will want to get the right vitamin D- D3, not D2. Many doctors prescribe D2. Prescription form of vitamin D may not be very effective or biologically active.

When you have your blood work done to check your vitamin D level, make sure it is the vitamin D 25 blood test for accuracy. You want your blood level at 45 to 60 ng/dl. If you find you are deficient, you may need as much as 5,000 to 10,000 IU a day for about three months or more. If you spend time in the sun from June through September, without sunscreen, you will most likely not need to supplement. Getting at least 10 to 15 minutes a few times a week in the summer keeps vitamin D levels at optimal range. Just remember too much sun exposure may lead to skin cancer.

3. Omega-3 Fatty Acids (EPA and DHA) – These are important fats known to support healthy brain function and protect our hearts. Take a tablespoon of a good fish oil from deep cold water. I like Carlson's Norwegian fish oil. It contains 1600 mg of omega-3s for just one teaspoon. It's lemon flavored, and I take it straight up. Chia and flax seeds are also great sources of omega-3. You can buy organic eggs with omega-3s as well.

4. Vitamin B12 – If you are eating mostly plants or a vegan diet, you will need to supplement with B12. Eating mostly plants, we decrease our risk of developing disease and increase our life expectancy, but we need an additional source of vitamin B12 because few plant sources contain this crucial vitamin. Even as we age, it gets harder to absorb B12 from our food, so a supplemental form of B12 can be a splendid thing.

Calcium Supplementation

The National Osteoporosis Foundation estimates that 54 million Americans are at risk for this bone-thinning disease. About half of all women over 50 will have a broken bone caused by osteoporosis. Consequently, doctors have been advising women to get 1,200 milligrams of calcium per day. Men have been advised to get 1,000 milligrams a day, or 1,200 milligrams for those over 70.

Common wisdom in the U.S. has been that drinking milk and supplementing with calcium helps prolong bone health, but the research is just not supporting this. In fact, the people who drink the most milk have more bone fractures than those who drink less. The British Medical Journal's online publication BMJ.com, supports U.S. health officials' latest findings that taking calcium supplements is not only a waste of time but could well be harmful. Perhaps the extra calcium is not strengthening our bones but building up in our arteries and kidneys and causing heart disease. The dairy industry would lead us to believe that osteoporosis is the result of too little calcium when, in actuality, one of the culprits is too much protein, the result of our animal-based diets. Consuming too much animal protein causes our bodies to pull calcium from our bones.

So what are we to do? Begin by reducing animal products from our diet or by completely eliminating them. Then, exercise! Exercise is our best bet for keeping bones strong and healthy. Weight-bearing exercises such as walking, running, tennis, weight lifting and dancing can strengthen our bones. Keep in mind that although swimming and cycling are great cardio workouts, they are not good weight-bearing exercise. Not only are weight-bearing exercises good for our bones, but, like any exercise, they keep our core strong and improve balance. Therefore, we are less likely to fall. I can't emphasize enough just how important exercise and movement are in protecting our health in the second half.

Reducing alcohol, animal protein, caffeine, sodas and sugar and avoiding smoking are also important. All of these things can weaken bones. I prefer to get my calcium from real food instead of supplements. Given the current research, I can't definitively say that this helps my bones either. However, the calcium-rich foods in the list below are all foods that are good in so many other ways that I'm recommending them anyway. Plus, if nothing else, there's always the "placebo effect." The placebo effect is a remarkable phenomenon in which a person's condition improves simply because that person has the expectation that it will.

Calcium in Non-Dairy Sources

Almonds – 1 oz. provides 80 mg of calcium, tames high blood pressure, promotes weight loss and cuts cholesterol (high in calories, so use in moderation).

Arugula – 1 cup contains 125 mg of calcium; 3 cups in salad has close to 400 mg.

Broccoli – 1 cup equals 180 mg.

Dried Figs – 2 dried figs have 55 mg of calcium (also high in fiber and iron).

Kale – 1 cup raw has 90 mg of calcium; a 3 ½ cup kale salad has more calcium than a glass of milk.

Oatmeal – steel cut oats are best with over 105 mg of calcium.

Oranges – 1 navel orange has 60 mg of calcium. Plus, oranges are loaded with

vitamin C.

Salmon – 3 oz. of canned salmon with bones has a whopping 181 mg of calcium, but you must eat the bones (they are soft, and you probably won't even know you ate them!)

Sardines – My favorite! A 3-oz. can in oil with bones equals 325 mg, or 33%, of our daily value of calcium.

Sesame Seeds – 1 oz. has 280 mg of calcium, almost as much as one glass of milk.

Soybeans – 1 cup boiled without salt is 261 mg of calcium.

Soymilk – 8 oz. has 300 mg of calcium, just as much as a glass of milk (take caution with soy if you are at risk for breast cancer or have had cancer).

Sunflower Seeds – 1 oz. has 50 mg of calcium.

Tofu – 1 serving (see package) has over 250 mg of calcium (I prefer sprouted organic tofu, which is easier to digest).

Turnip Greens – 1 cup boiled equals 200 mg of calcium.

White Beans – Just a half cup of white beans has close to 100 mg of calcium.

Magnesium Supplementation

Like calcium, magnesium is a critical mineral for the body. It is essential in regulating blood sugar levels, muscle and nerve functions and blood pressure and for making bone, protein and DNA. It is also one of the most critical nutrients for your cardiovascular health. Every cell in your body requires this trace mineral, and it is used to manufacture more than 300 enzymes, many of which are involved in energy production.

Magnesium has an important job in helping all the muscles in your body to relax. Calcium makes muscles contract. Magnesium and calcium work together to maintain normal heart rhythm by relaxing and contracting the heart muscle. Magnesium also keeps the calcium that is not absorbed by your bones from collecting in your arteries. Magnesium improves blood flow to the heart by opening up the blood vessels in your heart, arms, and legs. This crucial mineral is one you don't want to be deficient in.

It's not only your heart that good levels of magnesium help but also your mood and quality of sleep. Magnesium has natural tranquilizing properties. It is needed to produce seratonin and melatonin, important neurotransmitters.

According to one study, a deficiency in this nutrient makes us twice as likely to die as those with normal levels of magnesium. Magnesium deficiency is a huge problem with our standard American diet (or SAD). The reason we are so deficient is simple; we eat diets that contain almost no magnesium. Our diets are highly processed and refined, thanks to the bread, pasta, meat and dairy we consume. We also lose what little we do get by consuming excess alcohol, salt, coffee, and soft drinks as well as through sweat, parasites, diarrhea and even stress. A study in Kosovo reported that people who were under chronic stress because of the war there lost large amounts of magnesium in their urine. Magnesium can be poorly absorbed and easily lost from our bodies. We need a lot of it in our diet, along with enough vitamin B6, vitamin D, and selenium to get the amount of magnesium we need. All of these vitamins and minerals work together to keep us healthy.

The best way to get magnesium is through food rather than supplements. Natural sources of magnesium include leafy greens, kelp, avocado, tofu, brown rice, parsley, garlic, dulse, figs, dates, nuts, seeds, legumes, bananas and whole grains.

For the most part, foods high in dietary fiber are good sources of magnesium.

If you take a supplement, avoid magnesium carbonate, sulfate, gluconate, or oxide. These forms are inexpensive but do not absorb well. Use magnesium glycinate, or if constipated, use citrate. If you begin to have diarrhea, that means you are saturated with magnesium, and you just need to back off supplementation or switch to magnesium glycinate. *Those with kidney disease or heart disease should take magnesium under a doctor's supervision.

One of my favorite ways to increase magnesium is by taking a hot bath in two cups of Epsom salts (magnesium sulfate). The magnesium is absorbed through the skin while you soak for 20 to 25 minutes in water at about 105 degrees. I do this twice a week. It is my time to light some candles, read a good book and relax before bed. I sleep like a baby and you may, too. Remember, magnesium is the "relaxation mineral."

Killing Yourself Softly with Vegetable Oil?

Over the course of human evolution, man has made a dramatic change in the ratio of omega-6 to omega-3 fats that we consume. It may be this change as much as any other dietary factor that has contributed to our epidemic of modern disease. Our hunter-gatherer ancestors probably consumed omega-6 to omega-3 fats in a ratio of about 1-to-1. Today, estimates of that ratio range from an average of

10:1-20, to as high as 25-to-1 for some individuals. Not only that, but it is said that we Americans are getting almost 20 percent of our calories from a single food source, soybean oil, and almost 9 percent of those calories come from the omega-6 fat linoleic acid (LA). This change came in large part with the advent of the vegetable oil industry. The fatty acid ratio was also changed in the food we give to domestic livestock, which altered the fatty acid profile of the meat that we consume.

What does this matter to me, you might ask? Well, for us second-halfers it is certainly not good! Our high omega-6 intake is associated with an increase in inflammatory disease, which is pretty much all disease. The list includes:

- heart disease
- obesity
- type 2 diabetes
- IBS and inflammatory bowel disease
- metabolic syndrome
- macular degeneration
- rheumatoid arthritis
- cancer
- autoimmune diseases

(This is not a complete list, just the biggies!)

The big pharmaceutical companies know this effect of omega-6 on our bodies. That is why there are ibuprofen, aspirin, Tylenol, Aleve, etc. These drugs work to reduce inflammation in our bodies, but the same effect could be produced by limiting our intake of omega-6 fatty acids. The pharmaceutical companies don't want us to know this because there is big profit in all the pills we pop!

Pretty scary, isn't it? So what can I do, you ask? The first thing you can do is clean out your pantry. Throw away any safflower, sunflower, corn, canola, soy and peanut oils and never buy them again. I know they are cheap, but they will be the death of you! Stick with extra virgin olive oil and extra virgin coconut butter for cooking, dressings, and baking.

If you are going to eat beef, buy grass-fed beef. Why? Because grain-fed beef has "bad" fat and grass-fed beef is rich in omega-3s. Yes, it is more expensive, but you don't want to eat a lot of animal products, so you might as well eat the good stuff. Remember, you're eating more plants now! Also, limit how much you eat out. The bad oils are used at most restaurants because they are inexpensive. When you eat out, you might ask what oils are used in preparing your meal. It is very revealing.

The more omega-3 fat you eat, the less omega-6 will be available to your tissues to produce inflammation. Think of omega-6 as the flame, and omega-3 as the firefighter to put out the fire. A diet with a lot of omega-6 and not much omega-3 will turn up the inflammation in your body. Conversely, a lot of omega-3 and not too much omega-6 will reduce inflammation.

Our High Protein Diets Will Be The Death Of Us

"To be an environmentalist who happens to eat meat is like being a philanthropist who doesn't happen to give to charity."
-Howard Lyman

There are so many reasons to reduce or even eliminate animal products from our diets. There are the health argument, the environmental argument, and compassion for animals to be considered. Let's start with the health piece. Most Americans eat two times as much protein as they need. The result of this is a soaring rate of obesity, cancer and heart disease. What's more, our kidneys can barely keep up with the damage we are doing to them. They need to work overtime to break down protein and remove the waste. With all this abuse, our kidneys are at serious risk of stone development, of accelerated aging and even of failure.

It's not only that the kidneys suffer, but kidney problems go hand in hand with diabetes. Studies show that diets high in protein are associated with an increased risk of diabetes. Diabetes is a major risk factor for kidney disease. One study reveals that of 1,500 patients with diabetes, most had lost more than half of their kidney function due to a high intake of animal protein.

Want to lose weight? The American Cancer Society conducted a study over a ten-year period of nearly 80,000 people trying to lose weight. The people who ate meat three or more times a week gained much more weight than those who avoided meat and included more vegetables. Vegetarians are much more likely to be thin than their meat-eating counterparts states a study published in The Journal of Clinical Nutrition and The New England Journal of Medicine.

Many of us are concerned about getting Alzheimer's as we age. You might want to consider that diets high in saturated fat and cholesterol but low in fruits, vegetables, and fiber place us at an increased risk for Alzheimer's.

Of the approximately ten billion land animals slaughtered each year in America for our consumption, most of them come from huge factory farms. These factory farms that raise cows, pigs, chickens or veal calves do so in a very cramped space. Most live in pens and cages that are overcrowded, and many are not even able to turn around. Some never see the light of day. These poor animals live in an environment that is extremely stressful and unsanitary. To keep these animals alive in these horrible conditions, they are shot up with loads of antibiotics. When we ingest the flesh of these animals, we take in the antibiotics, the pesticides and the stress that they received. Factory farming is a very cruel industry, and although it can be heartbreaking, we need to understand where our food comes from. There are many good books and videos out there to learn more about this subject (see Recommended Reading, page 161).

In his book "Diet for a Poisoned Planet," David Steinman reports that of all the toxic chemicals found in food, 95 to 99 percent come from meat, dairy, fish and eggs. Animals store pesticides and other toxic stuff in their fat. We consume these carcinogens when we eat animals. A 1975 study by the Council on Environmental Quality showed 95 percent of our intake of DDT at that time came from dairy and meat products. DDT even at low levels has been linked to breast and other cancers, as well as male infertility.

Consuming meat in the quantities we do is impacting the environment on a global scale. Sometimes it feels as if there is nothing we can do to make a difference. The idea that the genie is already out of the bottle and things are too far gone, is simply not true. We all have the ability to make a huge difference not only for ourselves and the animals but also for our environment. We are the consumers, and it is our choices that impact this planet we call home.

There's never been a better time to eliminate meat from your diet. With a hugely growing population and so much land being used to raise livestock or the food to feed them, more and more land is required. Raising more animals means creating pastures to meet that demand. We are rapidly losing our forests in the U.S. to produce livestock feed, and 80 percent of the deforestation in the Amazon rainforest is attributed to beef production.

It is helpful to understand the impact of meat eaters by comparing the amount of land needed to produce meat with the amount needed to create plant protein. An acre of land is capable of providing 36 pounds of usable protein from meat per acre while the same amount of space can produce 224 pounds of protein from rice. Soybeans can produce 263 pounds of protein per acre. That's more than seven times the protein per acre than meat! Perhaps if we ate less meat and focused on eating more plants we could save our planet!

The scarcity of water all over the world is a real issue and will become an even bigger problem. The American West has been suffering from drought. With global warming, it is imperative that we turn our attention to conserving water. Domestic consumption comprises 10 percent of total freshwater usage and agriculture makes up 70 percent with a third of that going to produce grain for livestock. Yes, we should work harder to minimize our personal water usage, but we could have a much bigger impact by not eating meat.

Eating Out in the Second Half

My inner health coach is screaming, "Don't Eat Out! It Will Kill You!" OK, so maybe that's a little dramatic, but in reality, I am not straying that far from the truth. When we eat out, as I mentioned before, those nasty oils are going to be used. We must also remember that restaurants are in the business to make money. Corners are cut to make a profit, and a lot of salt and butter make everything taste good but also make it not so good for us. I may not be telling you anything you don't already know. Or, it could be that, like many of us, you enjoy going out so much you haven't given much thought to what happens in the kitchen. We get fed, and we don't have to do the work. What's not to love about that?

It seems most of us love to eat out these days. And we eat out a lot! Certainly, dining out wasn't the norm even forty or fifty years ago. Most people took their meals at home. It was the rare treat to eat out. For many, it's now the rare treat to eat in. Our obesity rates have risen right with our rates of eating out. A coincidence? I don't think so. A 2014 study published in the Journal of Public Health Nutrition found that eating out caused people to eat 200 more calories a day than when they cooked at home. I think that number may be much higher. Just an additional 200 extra calories a day would cause an approximate 20-pound gain in weight in just one year.

Eating out so often, we hardly realize how enormous the portions are. When I am working with clients, I suggest that they assume each meal out is going to contain two or three times the amount of calories that they need. And knowing full well most of them aren't going to quit eating out, I like to provide some strategies to help them eat out in a much healthier way. It can be done, but it takes a bit of work. But only in the beginning. Once you know what to do, you'll be amazingly good, like the "Vegan Cowboy," Howard Lyman. I just love his story!

Howard was a fourth generation cattle rancher, who, in his early 40s, was diagnosed with a tumor on his spine. He vowed to stop farming with chemicals if he survived his cancer. He was facing the prospect of being paralyzed. Howard survived the operation with no paralysis and started transforming his land into an organic farm. Years later, again with health concerns, he became a vegetarian and his health improved.

While making an appearance on "The Oprah Winfrey Show" in 1996, Howard spoke about his concerns over mad cow disease, and Oprah responded that Howard's remarks "just stopped me cold from eating another burger." Howard and Oprah were sued by a group of Texas cattlemen. They were both found not guilty of any wrongdoing.

Howard eventually became a vegan and vowed he would never eat another animal again. He co-authored the book "Mad Cowboy." In 1997, Howard was awarded the Peace Abbey Courage of Conscience

Award for his leadership in the animal rights movement. His story has been shared in two documentaries, "Peaceable Kingdom: The Journey Home" and "Veducated."

While home in Ellensburg, Washington, Howard put together a dining group of friends looking for good-tasting, healthy vegan meals. They struggled to find anywhere to eat a vegan meal. Howard went to the restaurants in town and told them that if they wanted the dining group's business, they would need to work on some offerings for them. What a great way to bring about change! Howard demonstrated how we can put our money where our mouth is. And if a cattle-ranching cowboy can eat nothing but plants, surely we can try to move in that direction, even if we begin by being meatless two or three days a week. You will be helping the earth, animals AND your body!

One of the reasons many of us eat out is that we are working so hard and eating out seems like the easiest and least stressful solution to finding nourishment. I would suggest that maybe it isn't as convenient as we think. First, we must drive to the restaurant, decide what to eat while we wait for the wait staff, place our order, wait for the food, eat our meal, wait for the bill and then drive home again. By the time we get home, much of the night is gone and we have likely spent hours on this endeavor. With a little planning, we could instead gather round the kitchen and make a much healthier meal in 30 minutes or less.

Ten Tips for Eating Out

Follow these simple rules, and you can enjoy an evening out without the risk to your health.

1. Be proactive. If you get to choose the restaurant, choose one with healthier fare. Do some research online. Use words such as local foods, healthy, organic, field to table, vegan, vegetarian, and hormone free, and you may just find a restaurant with a healthier awareness than most. Thankfully, I think the tide is slowly turning, and places like this are getting easier to find, particularly in the big cities. It's not quite as easy in smaller towns.

2. Don't arrive starving. Eat something light an hour or two before you go. Choose some carrot sticks and hummus or an apple with a tablespoon of almond butter.

3. Try to order a half portion or share an entrée with someone. If you can't do either, ask for half your order to be boxed up before it even comes out. You can eat it for lunch the next day.

4. Be the first to order. It helps to commit to your healthy choice rather than be influenced by someone else's bad choice that is way too alluring. I like to have a plan for how I will eat before I even get there.

5. While waiting, drink a glass of water before you eat anything. If you are choosing to have an alcoholic drink, have two glasses of water for every alcoholic drink you consume. Yes, I know you will have to make a trip to the potty!

6. Limit the alcohol (then you won't need so many trips to the potty). I find that being subtle about ordering club soda with lime keeps others from influencing what I drink. Have one drink if you must, but after that it's best to stick with water! If you are choosing a drink, try red wine, a wine spritzer, or a light beer. Try to avoid anything that has syrup added.

7. If they serve bread, don't eat it. Ask for some crudités to munch on while others are hitting the bread basket if they so desire.

8. When ordering, realize that you CAN make substitutions. In fact, you should! For example, if you are ordering a burger you might say, "No bun; can I get extra lettuce instead? No cheese, but can I add avocado? No fries; I would like steamed broccoli, and can you make sure they don't use any oils or butter when they steam it?" Ordering this way may cause you to feel a bit like Sally in "When Harry Met Sally," but it's up to you to protect your health.

9. When there is a choice of sides, opt for veggies and salad instead of potatoes, pasta or fried foods. You can also ask for salads with dressing, croutons or cheese on the side or eliminate these entirely.

10. Most importantly, enjoy your dining experience. Don't get stressed out when going out to eat or feel guilty for "being difficult" when you order.

And one last thought on eating out, don't go to a buffet! Golden Corral is not your friend. Try to avoid buffets at all times. If you are at a wedding or a meeting, you may have no choice. In this case, go through the line, choose the vegetables, the salad, and a small piece of meat. No bread, no croutons, no mac and cheese, no mashed potatoes and no dessert. Unless of course this is your 20 percent naughty day. If this is the case, pick either the dessert or the potatoes, but not both.

Does This Mean I Have to Entertain?

So now you know how to eat out. How about eating in? What the heck is wrong with your kitchen? Your dining room? Perhaps you have no culinary experience, or you just don't like to cook. If you can read, you can cook, AND you can entertain without all the stress.

I wouldn't have called entertaining stress free in my first half of life. When I was young, and my mother was entertaining, my three sisters and I ran around like a bunch of whirling dervishes. I am not kidding! Everything had to be perfect from polishing the silver to cleaning the house from A to Z. Not only did my mother whip that house into shape but she whipped us up into working as hard and fast as she did. Then the cooking would start, and boy did that seem like a lot of work. I will tell you that when company arrived everything was perfect.

Rapid housecleaning came in handy when Mom was out for the day, and we had to blow through that house in 15 minutes flat, cleaning up a whole collection of messes we had made. Or when the house was on the market, and a realtor wanted to show it in 30 minutes. But all this running around was quite stressful and did not make entertaining much fun. Needless to say, my husband and the husbands of the aforementioned sisters have no appreciation for this way of doing things. They probably think we are insane, and I have to tell you, our children don't like it any better.

Author and humorist Pat Wynn Brown taught me another way to entertain, and this is what I want to share with you (who says you can't teach an old dog new tricks?). Pat and her husband Steve often have two couples over for dinner on a weeknight. They serve a cocktail, salad, maybe an Irish stew and then some sherbet for dessert. It is so relaxed, inexpensive, and much easier than what I was always putting myself through. The best thing about being at Patty and Steve's was that the conversation was always lively and enjoyable, and weeknights felt like a weekend. They were the perfect hosts and although Patty was raised the same way I was, she had figured out this easy entertaining alternative before I did!

Every meal does not have to be labor intensive in order to share it with friends. One-pot meals are easy to prepare ahead. You also won't have the last-minute stress of everyone standing around in your kitchen talking to you as you are trying to remember what to do next.

People enjoy "eating in" at someone else's home. When you are the guest, you don't have to cook, and you don't have to clean up! Doing things in a simpler way may be just the strategy you need to entertain more and eat healthy dinners at home. The great thing about eating in is you have control over what goes into your food. As I mentioned earlier, many restaurants use oils like canola, peanut, and soy which are high in omega-6 fatty acids and often go rancid which can be toxic to the body. Restaurants also use a lot of salt and butter to make everything taste so good. Not the best for keeping our bodies healthy. Eating many of our meals out gets expensive too.

I still love to do dinner parties as my mother did with silver, crystal, beautiful settings and gourmet food, but I don't do this every time as I used to. It's just so much fun to invite interesting people over to share a simple meal and rich conversation. It's also not imperative that my house is perfectly picked up. I am still working on this part of the equation, I have to say. Old habits die hard!

My grandmother Audrey continued to cook until she was well into her 80s. She could manage a meal for 6 to 8 of us at that age without a problem. She loved doing it! I'm not sure why many second-halfers stop cooking. I suspect the convenience of eating out and feeling poorly from bad diets and lack of exercise are two of the culprits.

Recently, I asked an older friend if her MahJong group still took turns hosting lunch in their homes, and I was surprised by her response. She told me that some of the ladies pulled out their crystal and china for these occasions and others in the group had felt that they were "putting on the dog," so they put an end to that. Now they take their lunch at a restaurant. This was very perplexing to me because I like to do the same thing, and my motivation is to make everything beautiful. Is this what people would think if you did something special for them? I find this so sad! I am a believer in using the beautiful things you own for entertaining. That's why we have them. Some of my very best memories are eating at the homes of friends. One of my favorites is having dinner with Bill and Susan McDonough in their home on a summer evening. Bill is quite a gourmet cook, and their table was so beautiful with place settings I believe they bought in Italy. Their table was unique and colorful, a feast for the eyes. The food they served was as good as any gourmet restaurant's.

Another benefit of cooking is what it does for the brain. Cooking engages the brain in ways we need to engage it, especially as we age. The brain is like a muscle that must be exercised like the rest of our bodies. When we cook, we have more to show for our efforts than we would, say, with doing a crossword puzzle (which we know is good for the brain!). The trick is to keep meals simple, clean and healthy. We should have a repertoire of menus we can prepare in 30 minutes or less. More complicated recipes can be used for special occasions or just when we feel like making them.

Is Your Job Killing You?

Many of my clients tell me that they struggle to eat healthy while at work. At home, all is under control. They have cleaned the junk out of the pantry and are making healthy meals. Preparing healthy items for their lunch boxes, they have the best of intentions, but then it all goes awry. It seems as if every week it is someone's birthday and, of course, it would be rude not to share in their birthday cake, wouldn't it? The break room is full of junk food, and there are the jars of candy strategically placed throughout the office just calling your name. Then, there is the happy-hour team-building at the local bar. Here, we must bond with one another through drinking even though we said we weren't going to drink. The temptations are endless at work.

So, how do you combat the food pushers? First of all, remind yourself what you are trying to accomplish. What is your goal? Will you reach your goal eating all that stuff in the office? The answer is a resounding, "NO!" Second, think of these people as the enemy. I like to think of food pushers as enemy spies who are trying to poison me. It sounds funny but it works! It takes away my desire for whatever they're peddling. Next, avoid the break room, the cafeteria and the candy bowls. Find another route to move around the office if you have to. You can do this by bringing your lunch, water, snacks and coffee.

One of the best things to do is to try and change the culture in the office. When I am working with a company, I suggest changes such as celebrating a month's worth of birthdays on just one day — one cake or dessert to celebrate everyone who has a birthday that month. So instead of having 10 or 12 days of cakes and cupcakes, you have just one. I also work at replacing the vending machines with healthier choices, such as fruit, nuts and flavored waters. It does not have to be expensive to do this, and it works even better if you assign people to teams who then provide the healthy snacks for a week. Better choices emerge when the teams compete for the healthiest week of snacks. Having a vote and a little competition can go a long way!

Employers are looking at wellness programs as a way not only to help contain healthcare costs but also to help recruit and retain employees, especially in industries where it's tough to find people. I was working with a company that very much discouraged any sweets in the office. Each day, organic fruit and nuts were provided. The CEO is a woman who is very fit and health conscious. She is a shining example of living well in the second half. The office kitchen was warm and inviting, and I saw first-hand how the employees benefitted from this culture. It was certainly helpful to me as the on-site health coach that there wasn't all the temptation in the kitchen. I wish every employer were this committed to health!

There will always be people who try to sabotage your healthy choices, consciously or not. Remember the saying, "Misery loves company." You may hear comments like "Oh, you are just so disciplined!" or "We just enjoy food so much" or, my favorite, "I guess I'm just not that vain." Almost as if you had leprosy or something. Don't fall for it! There are those that know they need to work on their health but aren't doing so. Go ahead and feel the sting of their resentment and then continue becoming even more amazing! Give them something to talk about by getting healthy and gorgeous!

Pay Attention to How You Feel

When making any dietary changes, it's crucial to pay close attention to how you feel after eating certain foods. For many of my clients and for me, the white stuff may be tempting, but we know we don't feel good after eating it. I have experienced this myself. I call it the sugar fog. We get a bit dizzy, our eyesight gets worse and we feel edgy. This bad reaction is more pronounced now than when we were younger. Unfortunately, many of my clients have noticed how bad sugar makes them feel after eating, but out of habit, they keep eating it anyway. When we pay attention to what our bodies are telling us, it is easier to make the necessary changes.

Keeping a food journal can be the key to making the connection between the foods you eat and how you feel immediately or even two hours after eating. Note your energy level, your focus and how hungry you are a couple of hours after eating. Journaling has been shown to be a great tool for staying committed to a healthy lifestyle.

John, age 68, suffered a lot of inflammation and pain. While his arms and legs were thin, he was carrying some extra weight around the middle. I was concerned that this extra weight was causing his painful sciatica. I asked him to give up the white menace and evaluate if he felt better after doing so. He was very disciplined for two weeks, eating no flour or sugar. When I measured him two weeks later, he had lost an inch and a half but was complaining that his pants were falling down and he would have to buy new clothes. While most of us would be excited about that, he was annoyed because he had recently hired a wardrobe consultant and bought new clothes and now he had lost an inch and a half off his waist. I suggested he take his pants to the tailor and have them taken in. I asked him how the sciatica was, and he just stared at me for the longest time and then had an "aha!" moment. He realized he hadn't had any pain for quite a while! He had been in constant pain for months but hadn't even noticed when the pain went away. We need to learn to make the connection between what we eat and do and how we feel. It's just so easy in the busyness of life to miss these connections. Another reason a journal is good to keep!

Stoke the Fire

When we eat is as important as what we eat. And skipping meals DOES NOT equate to weight loss. Our bodies are amazing and geared towards survival. If we skip meals, our body will start to pack on the pounds assuming we are going into a time of scarcity. If we think of our metabolism like a fire, we can keep the fire burning and lose weight. Imagine a fire that just barely has embers. When we wake in the morning, we need to stoke that fire to get it going. If we skip breakfast, the fire continues to wane and our metabolism lowers. If we continually skip breakfast and wait to eat at lunch, the body assumes we are in starvation mode. So our lunch, that should burn as fuel, gets stored as fat in our body.

So, maybe you eat breakfast but don't eat a thing until lunch. The same thing can happen! Waiting 5 to 6 hours to eat again causes your blood sugar to plummet and lowers the fire of your metabolism. When your body finally gets the fuel it was looking for, it stores the food as fat instead of burning it as fuel. That's because the body has learned that your eating is inconsistent, and it doesn't know when it will get food again.

If you have eaten breakfast, by 10:30 or 11:00, you should be hungry again. Really hungry! And this is a good thing! It means your metabolism is working the way it should. This is when your body needs a snack. The snack keeps the fire stoked, and then you are not overly hungry and making poor choices for lunch. Some of the best snacks are a handful of walnuts or almonds. A piece of fruit with a few nuts is good as are some carrot sticks with hummus.

Lunch time rolls around and you should have a good sized lunch. Breakfast and lunch should be the largest meals of the day. That runs against our current culture of a very large dinner, but after dinner you don't need the same amount of fuel as you do after breakfast or lunch. Dinner should be the smallest meal of the day.

Mid-afternoon should find you starving. It's snack time again! If I am home I make a small protein shake or eat a few carrot sticks with some homemade hummus. For when I'm out, I keep ¼ cup measures of nuts or homemade trail mix in my car. Don't get caught unprepared! This is how our best laid plans fall apart and we drive through Dairy Queen for the parfait sundae with hot fudge, whipped cream and nuts. I know because this is exactly what I did one day last summer! The growling monster inside my tummy hijacked my best intentions.

By the time dinner comes, you should be able to control the portion size because you have stoked the fire all day. This should be the smallest meal of the day. If you are eating out, you can just assume it's going to be too much food. This is when you utilize the 10 tips for eating out. You won't overeat, and you'll have lunch for tomorrow.

What do Amazing People Eat for Lunch and Dinner?

For decades, lunch has been a sandwich filled with processed meats or peanut butter and jelly. For dinner, the star of our plates has been a big piece of meat surrounded by one vegetable and a starch of some sort. Unless you have been living in a cave, you probably know that there has been a big movement in food health to eat more plants. In fact, we have learned that we don't need that big piece of meat and processed meats aren't even good for us. So why are we still eating a sandwich for lunch and that big piece of meat for dinner? Old habits die hard, especially when we have grown up this way. For many of us, a sandwich is easy and it can remind us of our childhoods. Bread is a perfect vehicle to get that protein to our mouths.

Yes, we do need protein but not as much as we probably think we do. Too much protein can cause us to crave junk foods. It can also cause very serious health issues, such as gout.

I teach my clients to keep lunch simple. When eating out, order a green salad with as many veggies as you can get on it. Ask for olive oil and vinegar to dress the salad yourself (many dressings are full of bad oils, sugar and artificial ingredients). Greens need a little olive oil to help you digest the vitamins in them. If you don't like vinegar, ask for a lemon or lime to dress your salad. You can occasionally add a small piece of salmon, chicken or shrimp, but no larger than the palm of your hand. It can be helpful to have something warm in winter months, but this might be a vegetable or a bean soup in lieu of meat. During the hot summer months, it is good to keep much of your salad raw. When a salad feels too restrictive or boring, order the veggie burger with all the veggie toppings but ask them to hold the bun. I will even do this with an occasional organic beef burger or a bison burger and I really don't miss the bun, just the convenience of it as a delivery vehicle for my burger! I then ask for steamed broccoli as a side with my salad. This way I am getting another veggie, loads of calcium and something warm to satisfy me.

Whenever you can get home for lunch or bring a lunch, do so. By preparing your own lunch, you know what you are getting. Planning ahead is really important in this scenario so you don't end up eating something you will regret. Wash and chop organic veggies one day a week and buy lots of organic greens, like baby kale and baby spinach, that are prewashed and ready to go. It is a bit more expensive, but if you lead a busy life, this is definitely an easy way to get those glorious greens!

Make a great salad every day. This makes for a nutritious lunch. Add seeds like sesame, pumpkin and sunflower. Nuts such as walnuts, almonds and pecans will keep you satisfied with their healthy fats. Add some garbanzo beans, black beans or white beans to provide fiber and protein. Keeping these items handy will make lunch preparation very easy. You are only limited by your imagination!

Look for ways to add omega-3s and calcium to meals to keep bones strong (see Calcium in Nondairy Sources on page 48). I suggest trying canned sardines. They are very quick, they sit nicely on the shelf and they don't go bad for a very long time. Be sure you buy the sardines that have the bones included. You can throw together a great salad with arugula, baby kale or baby spinach, and veggies like cucumber, red radish, carrot and organic red pepper. Drain the olive oil or water off the sardines and put them in a small bowl. Then, break up a few gluten-free crackers like Mary's Gone Crackers and top the salad with this mixture. I have had clients that thought they hated sardines eat this meal on a regular basis. This tasty and nutritious meal can be assembled in less than 10 minutes, and it will keep you satisfied and lean.

I like canned wild salmon from Alaska as well. Yes, it can be eaten right out of the can without cooking! Toast one piece of Ezekial bread, put the salmon on and squeeze some lemon on top. Or, just eat plain with a salad or over brown rice.

Another healthy lunch option is baked falafel bites (see page 152) with tahini sauce, shredded carrots, pickle and cucumber, all wrapped in lettuce. Make the falafel bites ahead and then warm them just before assembling the wrap. They will keep in the refrigerator for five days.

One of the easiest ways to keep making good choices every day is to have a healthy repertoire of lunches that you love and to stick with them.

I like to keep dinners light. I think of dinner as a small piece of protein (think, the size of the palm of your hand), a green vegetable and a salad with veggies. I also prepare a vegan meal most nights. On these nights, my adorable, funny husband always asks where the pork chop is! I remind him that I would like to keep him around a while longer. For these meals, I love making brown rice in my rice cooker, beans, and all kinds of vegetables. You might sauté portobello mushrooms and steam some broccoli. Keeping it simple and clean is the best way to eat. When having a starch, use whole grains. You will digest these much easier if you don't eat them with meat.

My friend Kathleen reintroduced me to the cast iron skillet. She is single and regularly cooks for one. For about $10, she buys frozen wild salmon fillets at Trader Joe's and cooks them 4 to 5 minutes on each side in olive oil. She then pulls them out of the pan to keep warm and places sliced sweet potatoes in the skillet. In minutes, they are soft and ready to eat. She tosses a salad, and cleanup is a breeze, having used just one pan. She also has enough leftovers to take to work the next day. This is how she keeps eating healthy, all in 30 minutes or less and on a budget. Actually, she has found that she can get 4 servings from the $10 salmon. That's $2.50 per serving for wild caught salmon. Who says you can't eat healthy on a budget!

Alcohol

Alcohol is one of my favorite subjects as a coach because it is one of the biggest downfalls when it comes to weight loss and health. As I mentioned earlier, some things are difficult to say but need to be said. I probably don't have to tell you that when we drink, our defenses against overeating and eating unhealthy foods tend to go right out the window. Regarding moderation, this is another area in which many of us aren't actually "moderate" at all.

Alcohol is very enjoyable to share with friends, it helps us relax after a trying day, and over forty studies show a lower incidence of coronary heart disease associated with moderate drinking. Keep in mind, though, that these studies apply to alcohol "in moderation." So exactly what is drinking in moderation? Moderate drinking is one drink or less per day for women and two drinks or less per day for men. Sorry, ladies! But that is "the skinny" on moderation. Many of your doctors won't be telling you this because it is not too popular with most folks.

And boy, do I know just how unpopular this discussion can be with some clients and friends! Drinking is a subject on which I receive a whole lot of push-back. We love our alcohol. We have a hard time giving it up. We love how we feel after a couple of drinks, how it relaxes us and lowers our inhibitions. There are a myriad of problems associated with drinking more than we should. Alcohol has been found to increase fat around the waist. It also leads to a kind of withdrawal the day after consumption, which can then create a false sense of hunger. We sip away all of our best-laid plans to eat healthy and in moderation. Additionally, drinking more than a moderate amount of alcohol is toxic to our bodies. There is also the risk of alcoholism and damage to our liver. How many lives have we seen ruined because of alcohol addiction? Even when consumed in moderation, alcohol has been linked to a higher incidence of breast cancer and atrial fibrillation. If we want to get the best out of our bodies and minds, we need to drink less. There is just no getting around it.

Alcohol consumption should not be used as a crutch to go through the second half of our lives. I have seen too many people numbing themselves with alcohol night after night. Has drinking become a habit? Or, do people drink so they won't have to face their mortality? Some of us have become wine enthusiasts. Having built wine cellars, we collect wine, and now we feel compelled to consume all that wine. What I am addressing here are the social and cultural habits that develop as we age. As people age or even withdraw from their careers, they may increase their social drinking. Now, lunches out with friends include a cocktail. Five o'clock rolls around and, after a great round of golf, we have a beer. Dinner comes and is served with wine. Maybe you've started enjoying a Bloody Mary on the weekends. These scenarios play out every day in the lives of second-halfers.

I advise my clients to reduce slowly, one day at a time, the amount of alcohol they consume. It is much easier to do if you have a plan. If you drink a couple of drinks every day, take it down to one for women and two for men. I suggest looking ahead at your week and planning what days you might like a drink. Is there a birthday celebration, a date night, or just getting together with friends that you know will include alcohol? Have days that you don't drink any alcohol at all. When you do drink, learn to savor the drink you allow yourself. If you are at a function, ask for half a glass of alcohol. Take your time enjoying the drink while you socialize. Then, drink a sparkling water or two. Later, have that second half of wine. I have found that this keeps me hydrated and not feeling deprived. Having a plan like this in place makes it easier to be good. You can also choose to be with friends who don't drink as much as others, or you can set an example by not drinking at all. Can you be the life of the party without alcohol? Try it! It's not as hard as you might think. You'll feel and look a whole lot better than everyone else does the next day. If you still need more motivation, remember that drinking too much alcohol does not make for a beautiful face!

People who seriously reduce or even eliminate alcohol altogether find that they sleep a whole lot better. I have found many people doubt this because they often feel relaxed and a bit sleepy after drinking, but alcohol is a sleep disrupter. Many people who drink need to be medicated to sleep through the night. Try eliminating alcohol for a week or so and see how much better you sleep without it!

There are social drinkers, and there are those who are addicted. Many times the lines get blurred. A great litmus test is to go completely off alcohol for 30 days and see how you do. Taking a sabbatical from drinking is a wonderful way to check in with yourself.

Stop Dieting

Although trained in over 100 different dietary theories, I am not a fan of the latest fad diets. I watch people constantly fighting the battle of the bulge, trying this diet and that diet. Americans spend about $40 billion a year on weight-loss programs and products. It's big business! What we need to do is learn to make healthier choices and eat less. We must relearn how to eat, eliminate the processed foods that are killing us and increase nutrient-dense foods that are life-giving.

I have had clients remove the white menace and lose weight. I have had clients cut all their meals in half and lose weight. There are those who have chosen to eat only a plant-based diet and watch the pounds fall off. There is more than one way to skin a cat! What is most important is to realize that the changes we make are changes for life, not for a moment in time. We simply cannot lose the weight and promptly go back to our old habits and gain it all back. Well...I guess we can, which is what many of us do! Then, we begin the cycle all over again. Some give up altogether and return to living an unhealthy life.

If we keep our focus on the very simple truths outlined in this book, getting and staying healthy will be much easier for us. Our bodies do not like the gain-lose-gain-lose cycle that we keep repeating. Yo-yo dieting is hard on our internal organs, our skin and our general well-being. When we continue to fail in reaching our goals, we lose confidence in ourselves. Feeling stuck, we are often riddled with guilt that we aren't succeeding. Follow these simple truths consistently, and your life will be much juicier. You will have the time and energy to focus on more remarkable things.

---| **MOVE** |---

Exercise Does a Body (and an Employer) Good

The most wonderful thing about exercise is that it is the best way to keep aging, disease, depression and just about everything that ails us at bay! There is absolutely no denying the benefits of physical activity. When we move our bodies, we feel better, we look better, we sleep better, we have higher self-esteem and we can manage our weight.

Also, as we age, if we want to keep living independently we must be able to perform basic activities like dressing, cooking, moving, bathing and toileting. All of these basic activities require restoring or maintaining function. We need stability and strength. We get or keep these attributes through exercise. Knowing that 50 percent of the people who enter a nursing facility are dead within 6 months should be a great motivator! Why do they die so quickly? Just look around any nursing home, and you will see people sitting hour after hour. The highlight of the day is going to lunch and then to dinner. If they exercise at all, it's for just a few minutes. If we don't move our bodies, we cannot stay healthy. Moving our bodies is the key to longevity.

We need to exercise 6 days a week. Far too many of us don't come even close to this. The Centers for Disease Control and Prevention (CDC) estimates that 80 percent of American adults don't get even the recommended amount of exercise. The amount, recommended by the U.S. government is only 2.5 hours of moderate-intensity aerobic exercise each week, only one hour and 15 minutes of vigorous-intensity activity, or a combination of both.

What we know in reality is that we really need to exercise much more than 2.5 hours per week. So why are only 20 percent of us able to meet even the government's meager physical activity recommendations? The facts about the benefits of exercise are plentiful in our newspapers, in our magazines and on television. We can find a myriad of articles, images and workouts meant to encourage us to move. Yet, still, we don't.

The amount of education we have influences our exercise rates. College graduates make up 27 percent of those exercising, while people with less than a high school diploma make up only 12 percent of exercisers. Exercise is even less common if we are obese or overweight. The people least likely to engage in physical activity are those over age 65.

For some, the long hours spent at work make it difficult to fit in exercise. Some employers and communities are providing exercise engagement opportunities. Employers have been slowly stepping up preventative health. This is likely thanks to an incentive for employers to pony up more money to potentially cut healthcare costs later. One report states that employers have seen a 36 percent increase in healthcare costs over the past five years. Surprisingly, only about 18 percent of employers are offering on-site corporate fitness classes. High rates of obesity, diabetes and heart disease are some of the biggest drivers of our nation's healthcare costs, and they will continue to harm a company's productivity.

One study found that workers who spent 30 to 60 minutes of their lunch exercising, reported a boosted average performance rate of 15 percent. Workers in the study reported less post-lunch energy drain after exercising and, as a bonus, improvements in mood. Allowing employees to exercise at work may make perfect sense. We spend so many of our waking hours at work that the workplace can be the ideal place to exercise. Having this type of employee engagement not only supports the individual employee in achieving his or her healthy goals but also encourages others to follow suit. That's because being part of a community leads to the sharing of information and healthy choices. For employers, employee exercise has shown to decrease absenteeism and healthcare costs.

Do What You Love

We need to exercise. There is no getting around it. We can't eat our way out of doing it, we can't keep making excuses about why we aren't doing it and we can't keep putting it off until tomorrow. For many of us, that tomorrow never comes. But why?

Many people tell me they just don't like to exercise. One of my favorite clients tells me she has the couch potato gene! The funny thing is our bodies love it! We just have to get our brains to catch on! Have you ever had your dog refuse to go for a walk when you get out the leash? Or taken a child to the playground that didn't run and climb all over the place? Both animals and children instinctively know they need to move and, even better, they want to! Their brains just aren't all clogged up like ours with to-do lists, work and the other pleasures we seek.

I have found that when people make exercise a habit, like brushing their teeth, they become lifelong exercisers. Conversely, if they exercise in starts and stops, they tend to drop out and go longer periods before starting up again. Beginning any exercise program can seem like a daunting task, and at the beginning it is harder when you are deconditioned and finding yourself out of breath with just the simplest of exercise. The good news is, it gets so much better when we stick with it for a period of time. In as little as 2 weeks, we can see gains in our cardio health because blood volume increases after just 8 days of aerobic training. A larger blood volume increases your cardiac output and, therefore, your aerobic capacity. Weight training gains are a bit harder to measure that early on, but after 6 weeks of weight training at least twice a week, you will see changes. These changes are a great motivator to continue.

The key to moving your body is to do something you really love. Or a bunch of somethings. For those of us with ADD, we may need to mix things up and do lots of things to keep our interest. We may be jacks-of-all-trades and masters of none, but we are happy and engaged. For those of us who like to be really good at one thing, we may have one sport or mode of exercise we enjoy and we stick with that. And there are all those in between. What is important is that it doesn't matter our personality type. We just need to move our bodies, doing both cardio and weight-bearing exercise. There are so many choices available now. There is cycling, running, TRX, Pilates, dancing, yoga, Zumba, BODYPUMP, climbing, hiking, walking, etc. The choices are endless. We need to take an exercise inventory of what we enjoy and then do it.

So, how do we take a personal exercise inventory? I suggest you take some quiet time and reflect on what gets you excited. Think about the happiest times in your life when you were moving your body. Was it on the dance floor at a wedding? Was it hiking in the Grand Canyon? Cycling in Hilton Head? Taking a hot yoga class? Winning your neighborhood 5K? Or learning to surf in Biarritz? Write down those memories. Once you have done this, decide which mode of exercise is the closest to your best memories. Discover the thing that made you smile and laugh the most. If you don't have fun exercising, chances are you won't do it.

If your best memory was cycling in Hilton Head, you may enjoy a spinning class at a gym or getting a good road bike and hit the trails. Find the closest connection to what you really enjoy and you will be much more successful at staying with it. Staying with it is the key!

My friend John loves books. For years, John has walked an hour while listening to books on tape. John's wife Linda has a very serious and debilitating disease. Walking this way is good therapy for him and reduces his stress levels. The amazing thing is that he has stuck with it for eight years. I suggested to him that it was a two-for-one benefit. He says it's actually a four-for-one benefit. Walking a familiar neighborhood route, he gets in his daily exercise, he fills the time with great stories, he knows what is going on in the neighborhood and he's the built-in block watch. He is so well read. Just imagine how many great reads he has had in eight years! He also gets the audiobooks for free at his local library. How cool is that! This is exactly how to move in a way you enjoy.

Partner Up and Get In Shape

So, now that you know what mode of exercise you want to embark on, doing it with someone else can be so much more rewarding, especially in the beginning. Getting healthy and fit in community is one of the best paths to success in reaching our goals. Whether it's losing a few pounds or simply staying on track, having a partner has been proven to help. Once you are a specimen of physical fitness and in maintenance mode, you will find yourself moving without being prompted. In the meantime, I suggest you make a commitment to someone to keep you accountable. It could be a personal trainer, a friend, a coworker or a spouse. Before I was a personal trainer, I used a trainer twice a week. Steve was always inspiring and it didn't seem like work. I just had to show up and do what he told me for an hour.

Plus, we never stopped talking! I loved it and I got in really great shape. I can't say enough about having your own trainer. And not just because I am one. Personal trainers are required to have continuing education to maintain certification and are always learning new information. Many of them will come to your home, which makes it very easy to stay on track. You don't even need a home gym. A good trainer brings all kinds of portable equipment or uses your own body weight to work you over! Ask around for a good one or go to a reputable gym.

Even the most fit athletes have their exercise buddies. Personal trainers also work out together, sharing new ideas and moves. I personally love taking classes with others because I am a bit competitive and it makes me push myself in a good way. It can also become a wonderful social time for you to make new friends and keep the motivation to exercise. Isn't that what we need?

Over the years, I have enjoyed many different modes of exercise. I am one who needs to keep mixing things up or I get bored. I run, surf, cycle, kayak, hike, paddle board and row. While, so far, I have been rowing only on a machine, I am looking forward to rowing on the nearby river next summer. My new goal!

My friend Patty and I used to walk 6 miles a couple times a week. We walked very fast and talked the whole time. We never ran out of things to say. We decided it was free therapy! In that period of time, we managed to hash out everything going on in our lives that was good, bad or in between. We walked off those pounds along with any troubles!

I also trained with a friend when I ran my second marathon. It was a lot more fun to run and talk with someone than it was to run alone. Now, I run with my husband. We run together on a regular basis, and I always look forward to being with him. We also take trips that include a race, and it makes our travels all the more interesting. It is wonderful to have that to share together.

Get A Dog

Who needs exercise equipment when you have a furry friend? Your dog needs to get vigorous exercise at least 30 minutes a day and so do you. Why not do it together? Dogs love to walk; in fact, they demand it! Even if sometimes it's late at night when you would rather not go out. Studies show that humans find it harder to say no to a dog than to a person. Humans also come up with all kinds of excuses not to exercise. It's too cold or I'm too tired. Not so with dogs! Unless they are nearly on their deathbed, they will go every time.

One study showed that dogs were better companions than humans in terms of increasing fitness. The dogs in this study increased the walking speed of the humans by 28 percent, compared to just 4 percent among human walkers. There's a lot to be said for that.

Not only are dogs good for increasing the amount of time we walk, but they can also lower our blood pressure and generally improve happiness. Our canine companions love us unconditionally, and they never ask for money or tell us to take the trash out. My husband jokes that our daughters should never make us choose between them and the dog!! All kidding aside, dogs bring out the good in us.

Find Balance in Your Life

We have all heard time and again that life is about creating balance. This is literally true as we age. One of the first things to go as we age is our balance. It sneaks up on us; we may not even realize we've lost it until it's too late. If you are one of the unfortunate people who has suffered a fall or a broken bone, you know what I am talking about. We take our balance for granted, but we shouldn't. Our balance can begin to erode by the time we hit our 50s. It starts with a loss of strength in our legs and core, a decline in eyesight, and a decrease in our equilibrium which is known to happen with age.

Fear of falling is prevalent in our elderly and with good reason. It is estimated that about one-third of all seniors will slip and fall each year. The fall itself, with its potential for bruises, broken bones and even concussion, is painful and frightening. Then, there's the recovery period, which can be very lengthy. Not only that, but even after recovery, confidence in mobility begins to erode. This often leads the person to become more sedentary which then leads to even less balance and a decline in health.

You can work on improving your balance right now. Exercises focusing on balance can keep you steady on your feet, and you will reap big rewards later in life. It's much better to start now than after a fall. Having a good baseline while knowing your strengths and weaknesses can keep you confident and mobile. It doesn't require much time. Working on balance three times a week for just 10 to 15 minutes will restore your balance. In fact, you can always get your balance back! Here are a few exercises to get you started. Begin by keeping a stable chair or the wall within reach.

1. One-Legged Balance

    With feet together, pick up one foot. Hold for 10 seconds with eyes open, then closed. Switch feet and repeat for four reps on each foot.

2. Leg Swings

    Stand on your left leg and raise the right leg three to six inches off the floor. Holding arms at your sides, swing your right leg forward and backwards without letting the foot touch the floor. Remember to keep your torso erect. Switch legs and repeat. Now, swing one foot to the side and hold the opposite arm out to the side. Switch legs and repeat.

3. One-Legged Clock

    Place hands on hips, torso straight, head up, and balance on one leg. Imagine yourself a clock and point your arm overhead at 12, then at side to three, lower to six, cross body to end at nine. Try to keep your balance through all the moves. Switch to the opposite leg and arm and repeat.

4. Clock on an Unstable Surface

    Once the moves above are mastered, try them on a BOSU ballast ball or a balance disc. Be sure to stand near a wall, chair or ballet bar for safety. Now perform the one-legged clocks. It's more difficult now!

5. One-Legged Squat

    Stand with feet hip-distance apart. Place left foot out in front, just barely touching the floor and push your hips back and down as if sitting in a chair. Right knee is bent, eyes forward, chest upright and arms out front. Move up and down three to four times and then switch legs. Make sure you are pushing your bottom back and down so the knee does not go over the toe.

6. Single-Leg Dead Lift

   Balance on left foot, hold five- to 10-pound weight in hands. Suck in your abs, and bend forward at the hips with a flat back, reaching just in front of your left foot while right leg raises behind you for counterbalance. Keeping the buttocks tight as you return to the starting position, switch legs and repeat. Remember to keep the knee relaxed on standing leg and your back flat throughout the movement.

Sitting is Like Smoking?

If you ever needed another reason to get moving, here it is! The latest research shows that sitting for extended periods of time is just as harmful to your health as smoking. While you may have given up tobacco years ago, now it seems you must give up sitting as well. Weren't we supposed to be able to relax more as we got older? Didn't we imagine our golden years enjoying more time to sit and read, lounge in the rocking chair, knit or do needlepoint? So just what is wrong with sitting?

According to a recent study published in the Annals of Internal Medicine (January 2015), as you watch TV or even sit at your job, you increase your risk of cancer and other diseases. These increased risks are there even if you exercise every day. Another study even puts some precise numbers on the different types of cancer that might be associated with too much sitting around. For every two hours spent sitting in front of the computer or television, the average person raises his or her risk of colon cancer by 8 percent, endometrial cancer by 10 percent, and lung cancer by 6 percent. Not to mention that when you sit for long periods of time you stop breaking up fat in your bloodstream, and you begin accumulating fat in your liver, your heart, and your brain. You also get sleepy, gain weight and are generally much less healthy than when you're moving. Our bodies are built to move. We have 360 joints and 700 skeletal muscles, and our blood flow is based on movement.

So what do you do when your job requires long hours at a desk? When I work with people who spend long hours sitting, I suggest they find ways to stand up as much as possible each day. If you are deskbound, at the very least, stand for 2 minutes every 20 minutes. While standing may sound simple, your body will love you for it, and it brings on a positive physiological response. Your blood will flow better and you will breathe deeper while standing. If possible, take a walking break of 5 minutes every hour and get your blood flowing. When you are on the telephone, get up and walk around your office. Conduct "walking" meetings. Gather up your group and go outside and meet, or if the weather doesn't permit, walk around the conference room. It might seem a bit strange at first, but you will be protecting your health, and the bonus is, we are much more creative when moving.

It is helpful as you begin to make these changes to post a reminder in your office so you can stick with it. It takes some time to unlearn our old behaviors. I have clients who now have a timer on their desks that goes off every 45 minutes. They move a bit and then get back to their work. They have found that getting up and stretching provided feelings of well-being,, as does taking a short walk. They report fewer aches, pains and stress. Many are discovering they have become more creative by adding in more movement.

I have never spent much time sitting in an office. I have always been moving and going to see my clients. I felt the ugly truth of sitting for hours with the writing of this book. It was quite a revelation for me to discover how much my body reacted negatively after sitting for extended periods of time. Many times I found myself so engrossed in my writing that I didn't even realize three hours had gone by, and there I was still sitting at my computer. When I got up to move, my body ached, and my joints were stiff. I had to put into action exactly what I have asked clients to do. I put a timer on and got up to walk every 30 to 45 minutes. I also created my standing desk by placing my computer on a metal, three-tiered in-basket. It was just the right height for me to work.

And as for creativity, the best ideas for my writing came when I was running. Unfortunately, by the time I got home, I often could not remember what I had written in my head. I solved that problem by recording my thoughts on my smart phone. All it took was a few words to "jog" my memory! Movement makes for the best work!

There are increasing numbers of companies that are supplying standing desks or convertible desks. Some workplaces even have standing stations that workers share. For employees, this means improved health, and for employers, it can result in lower healthcare costs as well as employee attraction and retention. You might suggest standing desks if your company is open to new ideas. If you are the employer, the benefits of a standing desk are well documented. Many forward-thinking companies are starting to take this seriously and are taking steps to increase employee health and creativity.

If you work at home, you could stand and work at the kitchen counter for periods of time. Exercise balls can be implemented at the desk and even when watching television.

Standing and moving at work is a big shift in the way we have always done things. Change is difficult, but standing might be the best way to get the job done.

Carry Yourself Younger

As a child I was enrolled in my aunt Neva's charm school. My mother's younger sister was my idol. She was gorgeous and smart, and I wanted to be just like her. In her school we learned how to sit at table and which fork to use, and like Eliza Doolittle, we walked with books on our heads to improve our posture. These classes came at just the right time for my impressionable young self to soak in this practical knowledge; I never forgot what I learned.

Fast-forward to a decade later: as a professional model just barely tall enough to compete in the business, I dutifully remembered Aunt Neva's training. I was sure I could stretch my height a full inch taller just with good posture. To this day, friends will tease me about how I carry myself. The habit is very ingrained in me, but there was a time one summer that I noticed my posture had started to slip when

I was in my car, totally engrossed in my thoughts. I realized I was slumping over to the left; I had been doing this every time I got in my car! What had happened to me? Why was I doing this? I put a post-it in my car to make sure I was aware of my posture every time I got in my car. Eventually, I broke that bad habit! Good posture, however, is still something I have to work on, especially when I'm crouched over a mobile device, lost in thought, or sitting for long periods of time.

As we enter into the "second half," we still want to look good and feel good. Are we relegated to botox, fillers and face-lifts, destined to shovel our money over to doctors and beauty companies pedaling the fountain of youth? I think not! Embracing your age and carrying yourself with confidence and authority, whether you are young or old, is much more attractive than hiding behind a serum or scalpel. How we carry ourselves can impart an impression of old age or of youthfulness. How do you carry yourself? Do you walk slowly and round your shoulders, or do you skip like a child through your day?

We have so many temptations these days to ruin our postures and our good looks, from using mobile devices that throw our heads totally out of alignment, to sitting at a computer all day, to walking in high heels. Don't get me wrong; I love high heels! Nothing makes a woman look more elegant or beautiful than a high heel, when worn properly. If you want to walk in heels, make sure they are comfortable. I see young women looking like the Hunchback of Notre Dame because they are barely able to walk in their platform heels. That is not pretty! Perhaps even more problematic is the 70-year-old that breaks her ankle because she's still trying to wear stilettos. There is a middle ground that must be found.

Improving our posture takes some practice but is a whole lot cheaper than having a face-lift, and I think it reaps much better rewards. Good posture not only carries aesthetic value but also prevents medical problems. It affects how we perceive ourselves and how others perceive us. Body language plays a huge role in how we are perceived. One place to start is to stand with feet planted apart, hands on hips and the torso strong and long like Superwoman or Superman! Stand this way for 2 minutes each day. A study conducted in the Harvard business school by professor Amy Cuddy shows that holding this stance increases testosterone (the main sex hormone) and decreases cortisol (the stress hormone shown to increase belly fat). This power posing can really change our lives. In fact, powerful leaders have high testosterone and low cortisol levels. Professor Cuddy gave a great TED talk about this research, which I suggest watching. You can find it on YouTube.

When I walk, I try to imagine myself as that 12-year-old girl: full of life and energy with posture reaching towards the sky, carefree, in a bit of a hurry, and with a spring in my step. Walking this way makes me feel young. It turns out that growing up doesn't have to mean growing old!

Find Your Motivation

How do you find the motivation to exercise when you just don't feel like getting off your butt? When the couch sounds so much more alluring than going to the gym? Honestly, I have had these feelings myself. There has been many a time my husband has suggested we go for a run, but says that he doesn't really feel like it. We do it anyway.

Once we get started, those feelings dissipate. Almost everyone has these feelings, even professional athletes. There are a gazillion ways to motivate yourself to exercise. It's imperative to find what works for you.

The beginning of something new is always the hardest part. This is especially true with exercise. I say, "Fake it till you make it!" See yourself as strong, happy, fit and trim. Talk yourself strong, happy, fit and trim. Make sure the voice in your head is on your side and not working against you. Find the voice that says, "I can do this! I may have failed before, but not this time! I am getting stronger one day at a time. I am going to reach my goals! There is no waiting until tomorrow. Today is the day!" Not only fake it till you make it, but fake it until you become it! You can become an athlete.

I was never athletic as a child. As a matter of fact, I felt ashamed to be the last kid picked for any school team sport. Gym class was torture for me. I was little, I had no endurance, and I passed out every time I got overheated. Looking back, I think it was because of all the sugar I ate at that time. The Pop-Tarts and Carnation Instant Breakfast just did not serve me well. It wasn't until I was 22 years old that I started to think about getting fit. I bought "Jane Fonda's Workout Book." There was no video, just a big hardcover book with photos of Jane exercising. I did her exercises several days a week and it changed me. I started to feel better, I looked better, I slept better and, for the first time in my life, I felt like I could become strong and maybe even athletic. In my 30s, I also started running a bit.

I was forty years old when I learned that Oprah had run a full marathon. I had never run more than three or four miles at one time, but I thought if Oprah could do it, surely I could! I bought a book on marathon training, and then I told everyone I was going to run a marathon. For me, telling people I was going to do this held my running feet to the fire. Not only that, but I registered for a marathon out of state and booked the flight and the hotel room. There was no going back! I still remember that time so well. I was constantly amazed at myself. This body of mine could run 10 miles? Then 12? Then 18? With each gain in mileage, I felt amazing! And I was amazed at what my body could do. That the kid who was never chosen, the kid that no one wanted on their team, could do this? It blew me away! It was so exciting. And when I crossed the finish line there in Chicago, having run 26.2 miles, I felt as if I could do anything. It was one of the most empowering moments of my life.

The point of sharing my story is that if I can become an athlete, you can become an athlete. We must want it. We must fit it into our daily lives. We must overcome the voices in our heads that tell us we can't do it, that we aren't good enough. The point is we can do it, we are good enough! It is also never too late. If you don't believe me, check out Olga Kotelko's story below.

Olga is a 96-year-old track star. She was always active, but she didn't take up competing in track and field until the age of 77. Olga is the subject of the book, "What Makes Olga Run? The Mystery of the 90-Something Track Star and What She Can Teach Us About Living Longer, Happier Lives." This book examines her diet, fitness and personality and what we can learn from her about aging. She says that she chose to be a young-at-heart athlete instead of an old woman. Olga has won 750 gold medals and broken 26 world records. We all need inspiration, and Olga is absolutely inspiring! I won a race because of Olga. Let her inspire you too!

ath*lete
aTH,let/ noun
a person who is proficient in sports
and other forms of physical exercise.

Once you find your motivation, keep using it to keep yourself moving. Here are some of my favorite motivators.

1. Magazines – Fitness magazines with their fit models make me want to keep working. The articles are inspiring and I like to try new workout routines.

2. Books – The day before a 5K race in Key West, I had just finished reading the book I mentioned above about the 90-year-old track star. She motivated me to run faster, and I won for my age group! I figured if a woman who was 90 could sprint, so could I. Before the race I told my husband I was going to win, and he was very surprised when I did. I have not been known for speed! Endurance, yes; speed, no.

3. Cover Model – There is a girl who is a regular in the Athleta catalog. She is blonde, beautiful and strong. I tore out a page that featured her and kept it on my desk. I will never be six feet tall

or 20 again, but she motivates me. What I can do is get stronger every day and continue to build muscle and be athletic like she is. Find your cover and see if it works for you.

4. Set a Goal – I always have to have a goal. It may be the next marathon or a trip coming up. It may be preparing my body for a new athletic endeavor. Right now, I am training on a rowing machine in preparation for actual rowing on the water this spring. Since I will start as a novice, I don't want to be the weak link in a boat with other people. That's motivation!

5. After-the-Workout Memory – Remind yourself how you felt after your last workout. That sense of accomplishment, the rosy glow in your cheeks and the calories burned!

6. Adrenaline Rush – When I run or dance, I feel the rush of endorphins kicking in. I let that rush carry me through my workout.

7. Beach Vacation – OK, this may sound vain but it works for me! Nothing is quite so motivating as having to wear a swimsuit in front of other people. You may have given up swimwear in the second half, but don't you still want to wear skinny jeans? A sleeveless top? Do you want to have man boobs or old lady arms? Not me!

8. Fitting into my Clothes – It's bad enough that they keep changing fashion so we women have to continue buying more clothes, more shoes and more accessories (which we really do hate, right,

ladies?), but who wants to have to buy different sizes, too, or have to give up a favorite pair of pants?

9.   Workout Buddy – One of the best motivators ever!

10. Exercise Log – Writing your workouts down in a log helps to keep you on track. For whatever reason, writing it down is extremely important. I have found it provides a sense of accomplishment. Try this for a couple of weeks and see how it works for you. I think you may be as surprised as I was.

Recovery

The new buzz in the fitness world is all about recovery. Recovery from exercise is of vital importance for performance and continued gains in strength and endurance. The ability to recover permits continued robust performance at your next workout.

Rest and time spent not training (aka passive recovery), are different from active recovery, which refers to actions and techniques we use to repair our bodies after exercise. There are many ways to maximize recovery from exercise, and it doesn't always mean taking a day off. There is compelling research to suggest that active recovery is superior to passive recovery. Getting blood flow to the skeletal muscle bed promotes the resynthesis of C-reactive protein (CrP), glycogen stores, and the removal of protons. CrP is a substance produced in the liver and increases with tissue damage. I won't bore you with the science, but all of these factors aid in your recovery. One example of active recovery may be following a long, hard run or high-intensity aerobic workout with a yoga class the next day .

Recovery involves more than just muscle repair. We also need to recover our mental state, repair the nervous system, and replenish our hormones. There is a psychological benefit to daily exercise. Many people report that they feel better when they exercise every day. Moving the body can lift our spirits and mood.

Another thing to consider about active recovery is that some people find they stick to a healthier diet on the days they are physically active. Not only that, but with daily movement, we have the ability to burn calories, which can contribute to weight loss.

After exercise, the first thing to recover is our muscles because they get direct blood flow, but tendons, ligaments and bones get indirect blood flow and, therefore, take longer to recover. It is the tendons, ligaments and bones that become susceptible to overtraining. We don't need to be perfect concerning recovery, but we do need to give it our attention. So how do we recover?

Sleep (passive recovery) is our best way of recovering from exercise, and getting 7 to 8 hours a night is best. Drinking enough water is critical in restoring energy, performance and health. The best way to know if you are hydrated is to check your urine. If it is a pale yellow, you are probably hydrated; the darker it is, the less hydrated you are. Many people remember to hydrate during exercise, but do not hydrate in their downtime often enough. Eating nutritious foods is also critical for recovery. Food has the power to heal us or hurt us. If we are consuming nutrient dense real food, we will recover much more quickly.

Sitting after exercise is not helpful, and a bad posture will create all kinds of havoc with your workout schedule. Try standing at work as much as possible, and pay close attention to your posture. If you can sit on a stability ball while at work, do so. The ball will force you to use your core and sit in a better position. Make sure your chair is the correct height and is ergonomically correct for you.

We all know we need to stretch, but many of us just do not do it. We are so happy to get in our workout, finish and move on to something else that we tend to neglect this critical step in recovery. We need dynamic stretching while warming up and should save static stretching for after exercise when our muscles are still warm.

Self-myofascial release (SMR) is my favorite tool for recovery. My clients are finding relief and quicker recovery with its use as well. Tools for use include a foam roller and a lacrosse type ball. I love the new soft rollers much better than the hard ones of the past. The soft rollers achieve the same results but are much more forgiving and less uncomfortable than the hard ones. The idea is to massage your muscles. SMR improves range of motion and reduces stiffness. The ball is useful for rolling on bottoms of feet while standing and applying pressure as you roll it under the arch of your foot. It can also be used for shoulders, glutes and tight hips. On an active recovery day, try rolling over all the major muscle groups. Strive for 30 seconds on each major muscle group, avoiding the joints and bony areas. Be aware of the sore spots, spending some extra time with the ball on these spots. You can work out many a kink this way. Watch the pressure because your goal is to feel better after the rolling. Hiring someone for a few sessions in SMR is worth every penny if you have never tried it. The results are amazing, and my clients rave about it.

Yoga is a fantastic form of mobility that can be used every day for active recovery. Yoga typically works every joint in the body through a range of motion. The breath work in yoga is also good for lowering cortisol levels and blood pressure. With yoga, it is important to work in a range that is good for where your body is at this moment in time. It is not a competition. Yoga is about doing your best with your body. It doesn't matter what the person next to you can do. You will not get the full benefits of a yoga practice if you're comparing yourself to the perfect pose someone else just struck a couple of mats away. Finding a good yoga teacher and attending a class that matches your skill level are important.

Cycling is always good for an active recovery workout. While it is aerobic, you can regulate the intensity depending on your fitness level and training. Getting on your bike and being outdoors are also good for clearing your head. Be sure to wear a helmet to protect that head. If you don't have a bike or just don't feel comfortable on one, a stationary bike can work just as well for recovery days. You might even try a spinning class!

Walking will not only keep you burning calories on an easier recovery day, but it will also get you outside, which is excellent for increasing feelings of well-being. And short of sub-zero temperatures, ice or extremely high heat, there is absolutely no reason you can't get outside every day.

Tai Chi is perfect for second-halfers both for recovery and to reduce stress and anxiety. Tai Chi is an ancient Chinese tradition that involves a series of movements performed in a slow, focused manner, accompanied by deep breathing. The body is in constant, gentle motion flowing from one posture to the next. There are many different styles practiced, and Tai Chi provides something for everyone as it is low impact and puts minimal stress on muscles and joints. You can find Tai Chi classes in many communities or hire an instructor to teach you how to practice safely. Learning to use proper technique is important.

Heat, ice, and compression are still loyal aides in recovery when we have worked out hard. In particular, hard runs in marathon training or CrossFit competitions will find us needing these helpful tools.

We are all bio-individual, and recovery will vary from individual to individual depending on many factors, such as our fitness level, age and weight. For an ultra marathon runner, jogging on a recovery day at a slow pace may help with fitness goals. But for someone just beginning an exercise regimen, walking the day after weight training may be the best active recovery. For this person, doing too much may tax the body's ability to adapt to exercise. The goal here is to keep moving forward with gains in strength and endurance in the best modality for each.

Don't Be Selfish

We have all known people who don't exercise or make healthy choices with regard to eating. Maybe you are that person. I have always believed that everyone has the right to choose how they are going to live their lives. And in fact, yes, everyone does. But we all have a huge role to play in our own happiness, our own health and ultimately our own destiny. And we have a responsibility to those who care for us. What happens to them if we make poor choices? Don't we impact the ones we love? How about our society at large? Won't our poor choices be a drain on our economy?

The answer is a resounding yes! If you are married, is it fair to the spouse who has eaten healthy and exercised to now be confined to the home, caring for the partner who has never done any of this? How about something as simple as traveling with this partner? What if the healthy one had to spend a large part of his or her vacation helping the out-of-shape partner get around, pushing a wheelchair or being required to take frequent breaks before moving on? The choices of the one affect the other. How about the children trying to lead their own lives who now must care for an ailing parent?

Improving our health is a gift we can give to ourselves as well as to others. As we age, there are things that will inevitably happen with regard to our health that are totally out of our control. But we can and must do the things that are within our control. When we take care of our health, we may delay the onset or even prevent many diseases.

With more than half of all Americans suffering from one or more chronic diseases, the economic toll on society is enormous. It is estimated that these diseases' impact on the economy is $1.3 trillion annually. The following are seven of the most common chronic diseases: cancer, diabetes, hypertension, stroke, heart disease, pulmonary conditions and mental disorders. Many of these diseases are preventable with improved diet and exercise. How will we ever be valued as we age if we are a burden to our children and grandchildren, or to society at large? These are all issues that need to be addressed within our families and our nation. Even making modest improvements in our health can ease the burden on both our families and the economy.

Providing care for sick loved ones is essential and one of the most loving acts we can do for family and friends. It is a beautiful thing. It is truly a loving thing. For better or for worse, for richer, for poorer, in sickness and in health are part of our traditional wedding vows. These vows are important and meant to be honored, but we have an obligation to try for the "better" and the "health" part of those vows. We owe it not only to ourselves and our country, but also to our partner. Additionally, we will get to enjoy our children and grandchildren so much more if we make healthy strides.

This information can be hard to hear if you haven't been taking care of yourself. The reality is, it is not your fault. When the majority of the population is in the same boat, it is a cultural issue. With the advent of processed and convenient foods, we have damaged our health. With all of our labor saving devices, we have stopped moving our bodies as we should. The good news? No matter your age, or how long you have let yourself go, it is never too late to make improvements to your health. I will say it again. It is never too late! Our bodies are always seeking homeostasis, and every time we make good choices, our body will respond in a positive way. But this is where our free will comes in. We must make the choice to take care of ourselves. We only get one body and we need to honor it every day. To be amazing in the second half, you have to eat better and move your body!

The Something Else You Must Move

I'm just going to come right out and say it! It's POOP! Bowel movement is a subject my clients are often unsure about and want more information on. Some have trouble with regularity and are taking laxatives on a regular basis. A few think they go too often. Some have diarrhea more than occasionally. And others just want to know what it should look like. So, here's the scoop on poop!

The average person poops once a day. Exactly how often you poop is relative to the individual. We are all bio-individual so, of course, what is normal for one person will be different for another. Poop is waste, and we need to get rid of it. Some people will go after every meal. The average individual poops about 1 ounce of excrement for every 12 pounds of body weight. So if you weigh 160 pounds, you will probably produce just under a pound of poop per day. It's been said that Asians have more bowel movements than in the West because they eat a diet higher in fiber than we do. Many gastroenterologists agree that going anywhere from three times a day to three times a week falls in the normal range.

Many people report problems with regularity. They just have a hard time going. Often this is because they don't get enough fiber in their diet. Eating complex carbohydrates usually helps relieve this problem as does drinking more water. If you suffer from irregularity, drink warm water first thing in the morning. Every morning. Many of my clients have resolved this issue with just the addition of water in the morning instead of their coffee. For some, coffee helps with regularity. I do not recommend starting laxatives unless recommended by your doctor. Laxatives often cause more problems than they solve. Many of us become irregular when we travel or on weekends. Vacation and/or weekend irregularity is usually caused by a change in our usual habits of diet and exercise.

The quality of our poop is an indication of how well our digestive tract is working. If you are not pooping regularly, it could be that something in your body is not going right. It could be as simple as being dehydrated, or it could indicate a food allergy. A healthy poop is like a sausage or a snake, smooth and soft. If it has hard lumps that are hard to pass, that is considered constipation. If it has ragged edges and is mushy or liquid, it's diarrhea.

Many people report that they spend a lot of time in the bathroom trying to go. A healthy poop should only take a few minutes. If you are having to push or spending 30 minutes in the bathroom, this can lead to hemorrhoids, which is a very common ailment today with the modern diet. Increasing water and more fiber can help as well as elevating the feet about 8 to 10 inches while on the toilet. Our toilets are not designed the best for elimination, but simply using a small stool can be helpful. Many of my clients have found this very effective while on vacation when they are out of their routine.

Healthy gut flora is essential for good elimination. We have a ton of bacteria in our guts, and we need to keep adding in the good bugs. We can do this by adding fermented foods like raw sauerkraut, kimchi, miso and kefir. I like to get probiotics from food, but you can also buy a good quality probiotic in the refrigerated section of a trusted health food store. Make sure it has many different strains of bacteria and contains at least 5 billion cultures.

Eating more fat can help with constipation. Fat has a direct impact on peristalsis. These are the waves our bodies make to get rid of waste. Increasing fat can be very helpful for people who are constipated. Use healthy fats like coconut oil, olive oil, avocado oil and cod liver oil.

If you regularly have diarrhea, you might try taking a digestive enzyme that contains lipase. Lipase is the enzyme that helps digest healthy fats. It may be that you are not properly digesting the food you are eating. If diarrhea becomes chronic, you should see your doctor. Diarrhea can be caused by many things, including irritable bowel syndrome (IBS), inflammatory bowel disease, infection and malabsorption syndromes.

NOURISH

Think Yourself Younger

There are other places to look than the cosmetic and pharmaceutical industry for that fountain of youth. Just as we can move younger, we can also think ourselves younger. The mind is more powerful than we can ever imagine. Why is it that we now say things like, "Fifty is the new thirty?" Maybe it's because many 50-somethings seem more like 30-somethings these days. Think about a recent high school reunion. All your classmates are the same age, but some seem really old and some have hardly aged. The ones who seem really old aren't all overweight and not taking care of themselves; some have decided that they are old chronologically, and so their biological age decided to go along for the ride.

If you don't believe me, ask psychologist Ellen Langer. Professor Ellen Langer is a Harvard psychologist who has spent her entire career researching the power the mind has over our health. In 1981, Professor Langer recruited a group of men, all elderly, in their late 70s and 80s. These men were not told they would be in a study about ageing or even that they would participate in an experiment that would carry them back in time 20 years.

Through this experiment, Langer wanted to discover if she took the mind back 20 years, would the men's bodies show any changes? She put the men through physiological measurements before they started, a battery of cognitive and physical tests.

The men were split into two groups. They were driven to an old monastery in New Hampshire and dropped off. The first group stayed for one week and were asked to pretend they were young men again, living in the 1950s. Group number two arrived a week later, and were told to stay in the present but to reminisce about that time period. Both groups were surrounded with decor of the '50s. Lying around the monastery were old Life magazines, the Saturday Evening Post, black and white televisions and an old radio. They watched films from that period and had discussions about sports greats like Mickey Mantle and Floyd Patterson. They were glued to the radio listening to Royal Orbit win the 1959 Preakness.

Over the course of the week, the men started making their own meals. They made their own choices. They were never treated as if they were old or sick. Pretty soon, Professor Langer started seeing a difference in the men. She noticed they were walking faster and one man had even given up his cane.

At the end of the week she put them all through the same measurements she had done before arriving at the monastery. What she found were dramatic positive changes. Both groups were stronger and more flexible. Height, weight, posture, gait, hearing and vision had improved. Even their performance on intelligence tests had improved. Their joints became more flexible, and fingers were even less gnarled by arthritis. Furthermore, the first group of men who acted as if they really were back in 1959 showed more improvement than the second group.

Professor Langer says, "Wherever you put the mind, the body will follow. It's not our physical state that limits us; it is our mindset about our own limits, our perceptions, that draws the lines in the sand."

There are other experiments that demonstrate this very idea that our bodies will follow our minds. Nursing homes have found improvement in the moods of the elderly who listen to music from the era of their youth. As a personal trainer, I have played oldies while working with people who suffer from a lot of pain and have seen an improvement in their strength and mood during these training sessions.

Forgive

"God has been very good to me, for I never dwell upon anything wrong which a person has done, so as to remember it afterwards. If I do remember it, I always see some other virtue in that person."
-Saint Teresa of Avila

Possessing the ability to forgive is one of the healthiest and most healing things you can do for yourself. Yes, I mean yourself! Often, we believe that forgiveness is something we bestow on someone else who has wronged us in some way. We believe we are doing the other person an act of kindness. Certainly, to be forgiven is a blessed thing. But, to forgive is freeing.

There is something about living in the second half, which allows us, if we have grown up, to forgive in a way we didn't in the first decades of our lives. We have softened our once dualistic thinking. All is not black and white, good and evil. We have come to see human failings in a more practical and kinder light. Hopefully, by the second half, we have learned to bear with one another more fully. Our egos, now relegated to their proper place and not as easily shattered by others' actions or comments, allow us to forgive.

Our physical health will be in jeopardy if we don't have the ability to forgive. Carrying around anger can lead to higher blood pressure, the risk of heart attack, anxiety, depression and increased stress. Long-held resentments, felt for years, even decades, eat away at us. We have probably all known someone who felt wronged by a friend or a family member and never spoke to that person again. Witnessing this person's life, we see the repeated pattern of people coming and going from their world. They carry a constant pain with so much anger eating them alive. Many people harboring resentment come down with some fatal illness, have a stroke, become alcoholics, develop depression, or just end up bitter in old age.

I have found that some people are natural forgivers and some struggle terribly with forgiving. Can we learn to forgive? Of course we can. As I said before, as second-halfers we are much better at it in general, but if you find that there is someone you have not forgiven, it would be best to learn how. Deciding to forgive is the first step.

Forgiveness is a choice. Just knowing it is a gift we give ourselves makes it much easier. If there is someone who wronged you, maybe even as a child, that you can't go to, write down your forgiveness in a journal or even pray for that person.

In my late 30s, there was a woman I worked with in a volunteer role who hurt me terribly. I found myself thinking about her too often, dreading seeing her in public, and seething with resentment. Shortly after, I had gone on a dive trip to the Caribbean. When I dive, I am in another world watching the beautiful display of color and marine life under the sea. For me, it is a kind of meditation. I hardly use up the oxygen in my tank when I get in this state. All I can hear is my breathing; everything seems to slow down. Under the sea is where I was when I thought of this woman. It was the end of the dive, and I was under the boat using up what oxygen was left in my tank, and I sank to my knees on the sandy bottom and cried. I cried for the lost friendship; I cried for the hurt I felt and then I cried for her. Right there and then I made up my mind to forgive her. For everything that had happened! It was healing for me. I decided that going forward there would be nothing, absolutely NOTHING, done to me that I would not forgive. It was a momentous moment in my life and one I have never forgotten. Now, when I see this woman, there is no racing heart, no negative feelings, no avoidance, just a warm regard for another one of God's children. The emotional and physical burden is gone.

Not only must we forgive others, but we must also learn to forgive ourselves. For many people, this can be the hardest thing to do. If we have "lived" life, by the time we are in the second half, we have messed up along the way. The sting of regret, the pain of mistakes and our sins, have been the best teachers in our lives. We have all made mistakes, and as Kenny Chesney says in his song "You and Tequila," "It's always your favorite sins that do you in." We may have had a pattern of mishaps and been slow to catch on, but thankfully, by the second half, we have finally figured it out. These are the experiences that hopefully grew us into mature second-halfers. If you still struggle with forgiving yourself for anything in your past, I encourage you to work actively on this. Write a letter to yourself, spell out what is hard to forgive and then write that everything is forgivable. After you have written this letter, you can keep it, shred it or burn it. Then, let the thing (or things) go, once and for all.

Forgiveness is part of many spiritual practices and has been taught by religious teachers for thousands of years. As a woman of faith, I have finally grasped the truth, and that is, if God in all holiness, omniscience, wisdom, faithfulness and mercy can forgive me anything, who am I not to forgive others or even myself? Jesus demonstrated this forgiveness by making the sinner — the Roman centurion, the tax collector, the woman at the well and the thief on the cross — the heroes and heroines of his stories. Buddhism teaches the importance of a peaceful state of mind as well as a peaceful life. Buddhists believe that forgiveness is a critical step to achieving this peaceful state and that not forgiving causes suffering. Forgiveness is healing for all. If you doubt that, read Frederick's story.

Frederick Ndabaramiye is a Rwandan who lived through the genocide. He was just a teenager when he was ordered by a group of men to kill a bus load of people. When he refused, the genocidaires stripped him of his clothes and hacked off his arms. He survived because the ropes that bound him served as a tourniquet. Years later, he was to meet one of the men who killed the men, raped the women and left Frederick for dead. This man even acknowledged that he was the one who took Frederick's clothes. Frederick reached up, laid his arm on his, and looked into his eyes saying, "Yes. That was me, but I already forgive you." The man was speechless. Frederick said the huge weight he had been carrying around for so long was gone. And although he was frightened by the man for a few moments, he had freed himself from the hatred that held him trapped in the memories of that horrible day.

I have met with Frederick in Rwanda and at several events over the years. Frederick is one of the happiest people I have ever met. He is the co-founder of a community center that helps people to discover their purpose in spite of their circumstances. He is a shining example of what forgiveness is all about.

Sleep Yourself Younger

One of the common complaints I hear from my clients is about their struggle with sleep. These insomniacs either have trouble getting to sleep, or they are waking up and not able to fall back asleep. Sometimes they find themselves in the throes of work or personal problems as they lie in bed counting sheep. Many report that they feel tired during the day and have trouble concentrating due to the lack of sleep.

A bad night's sleep can have you feeling drained before you even have your breakfast smoothie. Sadly, almost one-third of Americans report that they lie awake at least a few nights a week. This needs to change. The quality of our sleep is essential to good health. Sleep deprivation is linked to high blood pressure, obesity, poor work performance, and a lack of energy for exercising, eating healthy and, well, fun!

There are many reasons for our inability to sleep. Too much stress and moving the body too little, or even too much, can interrupt sleep. Eating too much or too late at night can inhibit sleep as well.

If we want to slow down that biological clock, we must sleep enough hours each night and get the healing kind of sleep. Below are time-tested and client-tested tips for sleeping. If you want to sleep better, give them a try. You may have to try several or all of these tips, and you may need to combine a few on one night. Make it an adventure. Imagine you are a researcher looking for the cure for insomnia! I say this because I know it can be hard to get yourself to try new techniques. I have had many a friend or family member be unwilling to make these little tweaks, seemingly happy to keep complaining, and not sleeping.

1. Keep the bedroom for love making and sleep only (if no sleep issues, you may be able to disregard this tip.)

2. Soak in 2 cups of Epsom salts in a tub of very warm water for 20 minutes before hitting the sack (most of us are magnesium deficient, and magnesium is the relaxation mineral).

3. Create a relaxation ritual to do 30 to 60 minutes before bed. Meditate, drink a cup of chamomile tea, read, have a massage or massage yourself with a soft roller (I like the Melt roller).

4. Stay off your electronic devices like phones, iPads and computers for one hour before bedtime. This means no work emails, calls or studying.

5. As much as possible, keep bedtime the same each evening. When we do this, our bodies naturally know what's coming and get into the rhythm of sleep much more easily.

6. No caffeine. Even drinking iced tea or a diet cola at lunchtime may be keeping you awake. If you are a morning coffee drinker, stop at one or two cups and see if your sleep improves.

7. Turn off any blue-light sources an hour before bedtime. Blue-light sources are TVs, computers and cell phones. This may also mean covering your digital clock on the bedside table.

8. Skip the afternoon nap. You will find you sleep better at night. For that two or three o'clock plummet, go for a 10-minute walk, have a glass of ice water or meditate for 10 minutes. If you just can't live without that nap, make sure it's no longer than 20 minutes. Set a soft alarm to wake you in 20.

9. Hide the clock. Looking at the clock several times a night can make you anxious about getting enough sleep and keep you calculating how many hours you have left to make tomorrow a good day. Hide it in a drawer by the bed or just turn it completely around.

10. Check your thermostat. Most people do best with the room a bit on the cool side. 68 to 70 degrees makes for good sleeping.

11. Exercise 6 days a week but not too close to bedtime. Vigorous exercise should end 3 to 4 hours before your head hits the pillow.

12. Avoid alcohol. Alcohol is a huge sleep disrupter. It may make you sleepy at first, but after those effects wear off, you will be wide awake. If it doesn't wake you up, it may cause you to snore, at which time your spouse may send you to another bedroom!

13. Get Rover his own bed! Many people sleep with their pets, and while we love this, it may well be the thing keeping us from sleep. Pets can be retrained to sleep on their bed. I bought a very nice orthopedic bed for our lab, Oliver, which he has slept in from day one. We just never started the habit of letting him sleep in our bed. We have a little gate at the bedroom door that he could jump over, but it has been there since he was a puppy, so he never crosses it. We put his bed right outside our door, and he faithfully waits there every morning for us to get up. If you have an elderly pet that has always slept with you, this would probably not be feasible to do at this point, but it's something to keep in mind for the next pet in your life.

Guilt Free Self-Care

If you are the person who is always taking care of others, God bless you! If you are failing to take care of yourself, right now is the time to do so. Many of us feel guilty about taking time for ourselves and are just givers at heart. If we want to continue taking care of others, we must carve out time to nourish ourselves so we have the energy, the health and the joy to help others. Being a joyful giver is so much more attractive than being a martyr. Taking care of ourselves by eating healthy foods and exercising are two critical components of self-care, but there are additional methods to practice guilt-free self-care. And we need these things just as much as we need good food and exercise.

Feeling guilty for taking care of ourselves is an unproductive cycle of shame. As spiritual beings, we need creative outlets for happiness. As we did with exercise, we must find what speaks to us and brings a fullness to our lives. Guilt-free self-care is good for our health by lowering blood pressure, reducing stress and bringing joy to our lives.

Taking care of ourselves doesn't have to be expensive or even gobble up vast amounts of time. If you like to read, it can be as simple as carving out 30 minutes of time each day to read a good book. It might be lighting candles around your tub, soaking in sea salts and listening to relaxing music for 20 minutes. Perhaps it's going to the driving range and hitting some balls after a long day at work. Taking an art class might be just the creative outlet you need. Scheduling a massage once every two weeks or even once a month is something to look forward to. One of the most healing things we can do is getting out in nature, doing something as simple as going for a hike.

It doesn't matter what it is you do. What matters is having an awareness that you are doing something special for yourself. Say to yourself, "This is for me. This is my time, and this is what I love. Self-care is what feeds my soul." The awareness aspect of your self-care is an important component. Too often we are so busy and stressed that when we do something for ourselves, it doesn't even register because we didn't give it any awareness. With no awareness, just going through the motions, our brains may still be working on that project at work.

Scheduling guilt-free care is just as important as anything else you have on your to-do list. Decide each week what it is you are going to do to take care of yourself and then put it on your calendar as if it were an appointment with your CEO. After all, you are the CEO of your life, your health and your happiness.

Botox, Nose Hair, and Granny Panties

Growing old gracefully and embracing the changes that come is a beautiful thing. However, some personal things need attending to in the grooming department. Ladies may wear a lower heel and men Hush Puppies, but not everything should be let go of as we age. If we continue taking care of our grooming, even if it is different, we will feel younger. Feeling younger keeps us more youthful.

Women who let their hair go gray while sporting a great cut look good and men that don't color their hair or try a comb-over should be applauded. After all, it is our spirit that shines through and gives us our beauty.

There are plenty of people — in fact, millions of people — who like a little botox or filler to soften the lines and plump up a few spots that were once full. All you have to do is watch the evening news, and you can figure that out! It can take years off your life without much effort. While the idea of a facelift scares the heck out of me, I have had several friends who have had them, and they look good after some swelling and bruising and boatloads of money. Those who are happy with their results often exude a new confidence that perhaps helps them to be more social and move forward in their lives. If one plans to go this route, it is important to find someone who is a really good, board certified plastic surgeon. I do believe that a good diet, exercise and loving your life is much better than the pain, cost and risk of a facelift.

I have decided that one of the benefits of our dwindling eyesight is that we look damn good to ourselves and to others our age! The problem arises when we are around people much younger than ourselves. This is where the 10x magnification mirror comes in! I know it can be frightening to look in this mirror, but we need it to catch the nose, ear and chin hair that we can't see with the naked eye. This is essential because young people can see this with their naked eye even if second-halfers can't. And depending on how young they are, some of them will even tell you what they see, and this can be embarrassing.

Guys, don't forget to trim the eyebrows unless you are a character like the late Andy Rooney, and you like bushy eyebrows as your signature. Some people can carry this off but not many of us! Ladies, if you are lining your brows, this should be done with the 10x mirror in front of a window if you are going out in the daylight. We have all seen one too many women with brows drawn on that are frightening in the daylight.

And don't get me started with granny panties! OK, I'm going to talk about them anyway. Granny panties are not attractive. Remember the Bridget Jones movie where Bridget gets caught off guard with her granny panties on? How embarrassing was that! I could hardly watch; I was so embarrassed for her! Ladies, I can't tell you how many women I see who bend over and there at the top of their pants are granny panties! These panties are not attractive on anyone. Hightail it over to Victoria's Secret and get some pretty, colorful panties with lace and get rid of those things! You will feel much younger and prettier if you do this.

And men aren't getting off any easier! Tighty-whities every day are not attractive. Many men complain that their wives are not amorous any longer. Well, no wonder! Buy some colored briefs, or good-looking boxers for heaven's sake, even if they have superheroes on them. Just not the tighty-whities!

Freeing Other Care

While guilt-free self-care is needed, another healing thing we can do is to care for others. Volunteerism in the second half is such a wonderful way to take the focus off of ourselves and may even help us live longer. I like to think of Mother Teresa. Her heart was so engaged and full of love for the poor that we hardly even noticed how old she was. What we did notice was the work that she did. She never wanted anyone to die alone and without human touch. She labored for the salvation and sanctification of the poorest of the poor. Her Missionaries of Charity in Calcutta, and throughout India, did such loving work, and they carry on her work to this day. Mother Teresa lived to be 87 years old.

Studies show there is a reduced risk of mortality for those who volunteer or demonstrate helping behaviors. It is thought that as you overcome the fear of vulnerability in helping a stranger, your body releases a hormone called oxytocin. Oxytocin is a "compassion hormone," and it is splendid for your health. Oxytocin appears to reduce the stress hormone, cortisol, which as we know is not good for our organs and causes belly fat as well. When we even think about doing something good for someone else, the body releases dopamine, which is a feel-good chemical. Serotonin may also be released with these positive feelings. Serotonin is known to help alleviate depression. If you find yourself with chronic stress, other care can be a great relief to the body and can begin to heal you.

When we have a purpose other than taking care of ourselves, our little aches and pains don't take center stage. Taking the focus off of our issues while giving to others provides a healthy perspective we all can use as we age. Numerous studies show that when we are engaged in an ongoing volunteer role we enhance our immune system, we sleep better and we have better circulation. The University of Michigan's Institute for Social Research showed in one study that we have stronger feelings of personal satisfaction when we help others. You've heard of "runner's high"? Who knew there was also a "helper's high"?

Teach An Old Brain New Tricks

It was once thought that our brains started losing brain cells as we aged and there was nothing to be done about that. Just another "nail in the coffin" as we grew older. This assumption has now been challenged by recent studies showing that the brain is not in "park" but is still in "drive." In fact, the brain never stops changing.

One study followed London taxi drivers who must learn some 25,000 streets. Their brains changed much more than bus drivers' (who had fixed routes) because they were required to take different routes each day. The brain had to work at finding different locations, and therefore, more brain cells grew in the part of the brain associated with a knowledge of maps.

There is growing evidence that the aging brain is more malleable than was once thought. Neurogenesis, or brain plasticity, gives us the ability to keep forming new connections between brain cells and to alter function. Plasticity allows the brain to recover and restructure itself.

There is one caveat to all of this; we must keep learning new things as we age. It can be as simple as brushing our teeth with a different hand or writing with a different hand. The thing is, we must keep changing things up. We can't continue to have the same routine and do the same things day after day if we want increased mental capacity. The secret is to disorient and confuse our brains by switching things up on a regular basis. We can't rely on our old established ways of doing things. If you are the kind of person who loves learning new things, and then gets bored, only to move on to something else, your jack-of-all-trades mentality may very well be good for your brain. But, if you like your routine the same, day in and day out, you might want to rethink.

Plasticity can be improved by learning a new language, learning mathematics, taking dance lessons or even practicing identifying birds by their songs. Pushing and nourishing your brain can be as simple as taking a different route to work. Get out of your comfort zone by traveling to exotic places, navigating in unfamiliar terrain and learning new foods. Anything that challenges the brain's status quo will give you a complexity you didn't have before and keep your brain developing in the second half. In other words, get off autopilot.

Staying socially active requires a lot of effort for the brain and is especially useful as we age. Contributing to a conversation and following what is being said requires mental prowess. Many of us are content to stay in our comfort zones with the same social group. It can be of benefit to go to functions that require us to engage with people we have never met before. When we have no previous connection to someone, our brains must search for new ways to connect at a social level. Haven't we all felt the discomfort of being at a party where we hardly knew anyone? Embracing this challenge is the very thing we should be doing to keep our brains fit. One of the best predictors of healthy second-halfers is a busy social life.

Working crossword puzzles and doing Sudoku are familiar ways to work out your brain. These brain games target very specific cognitive abilities, but they don't carry over into real life. If you want to improve your brain, in addition to learning new things and changing routines, then bolster your cardiovascular fitness. Whether it's walking, running or rowing, sweating is what your brain needs the most. These exercises will help you with driving, crossing a busy street and improving balance. For building cognition, a crossword puzzle is a slingshot, and exercise is the rocket launcher.

Say Yes When You Want To Say No

Staying connected socially is crucial as we age. Sometimes, we just may not feel like going out with friends or going dancing. This is when we need to push ourselves to get out! It is our social connections that help keep us young, happy and living longer. If you were the life of the party in your 20s, remaining social might not be as easy as you grow older. Career changes, retirement, illness, pain and death can take away close friends. And as we age we will lose even more of our friends.

In a Finnish study, it was revealed that social activity helps to maintain mobility, and this decreases mortality risk. Perhaps mobility improved because many social activities include physical activity. Mobility is essential if you want to stay social. If we lose our ability to get around, we will likely become isolated and disconnected. Odds are we will become depressed if we are not mobile. This is not where we want to "go" in our later years. The study revealed that participating in things such as cultural activities, dancing, traveling or fitness in groups gave individuals a sense of belonging. These collective activities ingrained a sense of being liked, accepted and worthy of love — all of which are fundamental to well-being at every stage of life.

It takes a bit of work to stay connected with others as we age, but the effort can pay off big rewards. Good cognitive function and a lack of depression are just two of those payoffs. If your group starts to dwindle, start making new friends. Join a gym, a book club, a Bible study, a tennis group, etc. Do what you love and you'll meet others in the process. Make friends that are not only your age but younger than you as well. My mother-in-law had a wonderful circle of friends, but they were all about the same age, and when she was 95, she was the "last woman standing." There wasn't one close friend left. For women, it's also important to have a good group of girlfriends because as we know, the ladies tend to outlive the guys. And when that loving spouse is gone, you'll want to reach to your girlfriends for companionship, or you'll have to train a new boyfriend!!

We should make sure we are with at least one person each and every day. Being alone day after day is not healthy, and phone or email contact does not count. Physically being with someone is the essential thing. Exercising and volunteerism make perfect opportunities to not only stay mobile but also to connect socially.

Embrace Each Birthday

I always feel a bit sad when I hear that someone dreads an upcoming birthday. I wish everyone could be happy at whatever age they are. I'm not saying that I'm in a rush to be 90, but I want to enjoy each step along the way. Living another day and seeing another birthday is a privilege. It is important for us to live each day fully, to live in the moment, but also to be excited about what lies ahead.

As children, we look forward to turning 13, when we are finally teenagers. Then we long to be eighteen, when we become adults. Twenty-one is a biggie, being the legal age to buy a drink. At 21, we finally felt like adults who had arrived. It seems as if after the age of 21, many of us believe there is not a birthday worth looking forward to. Everything is surely downhill from there. I challenge you to think of a time when you thought 30 was old. As the age of 30 arrived, you realized it wasn't old at all. The truth is our spirits never age. That is the beautiful thing about our spirit. If we are living meaningful lives, we should embrace each and every birthday.

While writing this, I was reminded by a friend of the book "Tuesdays With Morrie." I remembered what a great read it was and the poignant lessons I learned from it. Morrie Schwartz was author Mitch Albom's former professor and mentor. Morrie had been diagnosed with ALS, Lou Gehrig's disease. Mitch, a sports journalist writing for the Detroit Free Press, sought and found his former professor. Visiting Morrie every Tuesday at the end of Morrie's life, Mitch learned valuable lessons about life and death. Mitch asked Morrie many meaningful questions in the brief time he spent with him. One was, "Weren't you ever afraid to grow old?" Morrie replied, "Mitch, I embrace aging. If you stayed at twenty-two, you'd always be as ignorant as you were at twenty-two. It's more than the negative that you're going to die; it's also the positive that you understand you're going to die, and that you live a better life because of it." Mitch replies, "Yes, but if aging were so valuable, why do people always say, 'Oh if I were young again.'" Morrie responds that that reflects unsatisfied and unfulfilled lives. "Lives that haven't found meaning. Because if you've found meaning in your life, you don't want to go back. You want to go forward. You want to see more, do more."

As Morrie advised, if we keep battling against getting older, we will always be unhappy because it's going to happen anyway. It is a fact that we are all eventually going to die. It is as much a part of life as birth. Continually battling against aging is a waste of time. Accepting and loving ourselves at any age is a beautiful thing. Learn to celebrate yourself and all that you've become with every birthday. With age, we should be much wiser, kinder and a whole lot more interesting than we were at 30.

If, as Morrie said, you feel unfulfilled, it's never too late to find meaning. We are never too old to contribute our gifts to the world. We all have gifts to give. Get yours out, shake it off and share it. Morrie shared his gifts through the wisdom he imparted from his bed in a few months of Tuesdays. Wisdom that will never be forgotten, a gift for anyone to take.

Laugh

One of the best things about life in the second half is the ability to laugh, at not only ourselves but many things. It sounds so cliché to say that laughter is the best medicine, but it is.

It seems as if we are not as easily wounded when we are the subject of some friendly ribbing in the second half. We know our weaknesses and our strengths. We aren't as interested in hiding our little peculiarities as we once were. We can laugh at ourselves now.

This is a good thing. We don't have to keep putting up that "perfect" facade we felt we needed when we were younger. And surrounding ourselves with people who make us laugh is a whole lot easier than spending time with the Debbie Downers in our life.

Laughter is one of the biggest reasons I married my husband. He is hysterical. It is a God-given gift. I admire that in him, and although I can't carry a joke in a bucket, somebody has to be the straight man! I reap the health benefits of his gift. We all know people who make us "bust a gut." Spend more time with those people; they are healers.

If you want to laugh more, turn off CNN and Fox News. My friends often complain about their parents who have the news on 24/7. Seeing the news all day will certainly not help in the laughter department. In fact, Dr. Andrew Weil suggests taking a news fast by turning off the tube for a few days or even a week. He believes that periodic breaks from the news promote mental calm and help to renew your spirit. Quite a few studies suggest that the images of violence, death and disaster can promote undesirable changes in mood and can lead to anxiety, sadness and depression — all of which can impact our health in a negative way.

Be selective where you spend your leisure time. If you like to go to the movies, you may want to choose a romantic comedy instead of the latest apocalyptic film that makes your heart race and sends you running home to change your pants. Spend time with friends that are upbeat, optimistic and full of joy. These people can remind us to keep moving forward with joy and embrace all that life throws at us. I often hear people complaining about their friends, their volunteer work or even their church. Find joy and laughter in all the areas of your life or make a change. Life is way too short! Carefully guarding our leisure time can lead to better coping skills, stress reduction and more laughter.

If we can laugh at our memory (or lack thereof), at each other and at our life, that life will be a whole lot richer and certainly more fun.

Love

"Love is deaf...you can't just tell someone you love them. You have to show it."

-Unknown

Focusing on love should be our primary occupation in the second half. Love is not a noun; it is a verb. Love requires action. A loving heart is one of the most healing things we can possess. We can eat all the right foods, take supplements and exercise, but it is our attitude and heartfelt emotions that can have the most profound effect on our health. When we can look upon everyone in a loving way, it brings lower cortisol levels, lower blood pressure, a healthier immune system and more feel-good hormones.

Whenever we touch someone (a friend, a lover), our brain releases the so-called love hormone, oxytocin. High levels of this hormone can boost libido, decrease stress, lower blood pressure and heighten trust. Hugging someone or kissing with your partner can boost your levels of oxytocin. Even thinking of hugging someone we love can increase the feel good hormones, too. We humans need touch all through life for good health. From the tiniest babies to the very oldest of old, hugging, kissing, cuddling and touching are essential.

For partners, the second half should be a time that allows us to disconnect from all of our daily distractions (TV, cell phones, Facebook) and snuggle up with one another. Keeping a close and loving connection makes us happier, healthier and more satisfied with our lives. Love your partner enough and be vulnerable enough to tell him or her what it is you need. Keep the love bond going. You will live longer. If your relationship is strained or because of children you haven't spent enough time with one another, now is the time to invest in the relationship. Rediscover what you loved about this person in the beginning, what made your heart race. It is there somewhere; you just have to find it again. Crabbing at one another in your golden years is not attractive or health promoting.

If you have held back in handing out hugs or in the public-display-of-affection department for most of your life, this is a good time to let go and "love-up" everyone around you. People like a genuine hugger. Don't be one of those insincere A-frame huggers! Hug like you mean it. You could be hugging that person on the last day of their life or even your own! My friend Marilyn is a great hugger, probably the best there is. When she hugs you, she grabs you and squeezes you tight. I'm not the only one who says this about her. It's a gift of love she imparts like no one else. Try it and see how people react and also how good it makes you feel!

My friend Adriana is from Brazil and she loves-up everyone around her. The first time she grabbed me and planted a big kiss on my cheek, I melted. I was not used to such a display of affection from a girlfriend. Americans don't tend to be that exuberant, but it made me feel wonderful. She had just recently moved to my city, and I was one of her first friends. Adriana said that I didn't need her for a friend because I already had lots of friends. She was so wrong about that; I needed someone like her to show me that a loving exuberance is something we all need. It is interesting that in the U.S., we have a term for showing affection in public ("PDA"). There is no word for this in Portuguese because this type of behavior happens all the time in Brazil; it's expected.

Loving-up those around you is healing not only for the recipient but also for yourself. Our world needs a lot more love, and we second-halfers can dish it out. There is so much pain and suffering in the world that is out of our control. Loving those around us who we encounter each and every day is something we can control.

And don't just reserve these feelings for family and friends. We can love-up the homeless man on the street by asking him what he needs and holding his hand. We can hold the door for a mother with a cranky toddler, smile and say hello to a stranger on the elevator, or visit an elderly widow who is all alone. There are just endless ways to spread the love.

Spirituality

*"Since many of you do not belong to the Catholic Church and
others are non-believers, from the bottom of my heart I give
this silent blessing to each and every one of you, respecting the
conscience of each one of you but knowing that each one of you is
a child of God."*

-Pope Francis

Spirituality means different things to all of us. Spirituality is a way to find comfort, peace and hope in our lives. For some of us, we participate in organized religion. We go to church, synagogue, a mosque, and so on. Some people find spirituality through art, music or nature. Others find it in the way they live their lives, in their values and principles.

A correlation has been found between being a churchgoer and living longer. The longevity factor is most pronounced for those who have never smoked, go to church on a weekly basis, have at least twelve years of education and are married. There is no scientific evidence yet that it's the practice of faith that results in longevity. Perhaps religious people are the type who would practice healthy behaviors regardless of their faith. Either way, it is an intriguing finding.

Beyond possibly extending life, there are many beneficial spiritual aspects to consider. Places of worship create a kind of meditative atmosphere that can lower stress levels. Giving thanks is part of many of these services, and we know that gratitude is significant to our mental health. The preaching of love, forgiveness, and hope fosters a positive outlook on life and is good for promoting emotional health. The religions that incorporate confession, such as Roman Catholicism, may help people release emotional burdens.

Many hospice nurses say their patients of faith make the transition from this life to the next more easily than those with no faith. Hospice nurse Trudy Harris speaks of a repeated pattern she experiences in her work. The closer her patients come to dying, the more their eyes and spirits seem to open to a reality she could only dimly glimpse. Her patients recount not just visits from absent loved ones but an extraordinary awareness of God's presence. Sins they had agonized over for years suddenly felt forgiven. Grievances they'd spent a lifetime nurturing vanished in a rush of reconciliation. Even unbelievers yearned for God. Thanks to Trudy's patients, she says she has been able to catch glimpses of heaven while here on earth.

I was blessed to have had all four of my grandparents into early adulthood. While in my 20s, I spent a lot of time visiting my aging grandmothers (at this time, just the grandmothers were living). It brought them such joy to see my daughters, their great-grand-daughters. They just lit up whenever I came for a visit. I remember vividly my father's mother, Audrey, saying that she couldn't wait to see Jesus' face. She was in her 90s at this time. When you are in your 20s, Jesus' face is not exactly what you think you want to see. I would guess that holds true for most 20-somethings, except the saints, one of which I am not! What is true for me now, is that in the second half, I understand what she meant. She had lived her life well. She was content. She had a love for Jesus, and her faith gave her strength.

I no longer have the same fears I had in my 20s. My faith has grown and given me a peace and comfort I didn't have then. Now, I can say the same thing. As a Christian, I do look forward to seeing Jesus' face. Author and priest Father Richard Rohr explains that we feel a longing, or "homesickness." I believe that this is what my grandmother was feeling.

It is often said that we are spiritual beings in a material world. We know that there is a positive connection to our health when we have a spiritual life. If you want to improve your spiritual health, there are some things you can do. First, identify the things in your life that give you a sense of peace, comfort, strength, love and a feeling of connectedness. Then, set aside time each day to practice the things that you have identified. It may be praying, meditating, getting out in nature, reading the Bible, or attending religious services. Taking the time to deepen our spiritual life can bring us comfort as we go through this second half. If you feel a longing or emptiness that can not be filled with material things or worldly pleasures, perhaps God is what your heart is seeking.

Hopefully, with age, we have become mature, we have become whole, and we see with loving eyes the things that matter the most. There is wisdom along with contentment that can come to us in this amazing second half.

RECIPES

While this is not a cookbook, I did want to share with you a few of my favorite recipes that are hits with almost everyone. These recipes are proof that you can eat healthy and still enjoy eating.

Appetizers

Sprouted Quinoa Tabbouleh

Tabbouleh is a yummy Lebanese dish full of greens, herbs and spices. This recipe has been adapted to make it gluten free but is still really good! I like to take to a potluck so I'm not tempted to eat junk. It is also my choice for a party appetizer served with veggies and crackers.

Allow time to sprout the quinoa 24 hours in advance. I soak my quinoa overnight, rinse in the morning, and prepare before dinner or going out.

Serves 6

½ cup quinoa
½ cup fresh mint, chopped
½ cup fresh flat-leaf parsley, chopped
1 cup cucumber, diced
2 medium tomatoes, cut into ¼-inch pieces
2 tablespoons extra virgin olive oil
2 garlic cloves, minced
¼ cup lemon juice
Sea salt to taste

Sprouting Quinoa

Rinse quinoa in fine mesh strainer and place in bowl with enough water to cover. Allow quinoa to absorb water (about 4 hours). Once water is absorbed, place quinoa back in strainer, rinse, set on plate and leave on counter. Rinse 2 more times throughout the day. *Don't forget to rinse! Quinoa will sprout/germinate within 24 hours.

Assembling Salad

In large bowl, combine sprouted quinoa with remaining ingredients. Serve chilled or at room temperature.

Vidalia Onion Dip

This dip is a real hit at parties and people don't even know it's a healthier choice. You can do both cheeses as vegan choices or use real parmesan cheese for the top if you want to ease into this vegan option.

Serves 16

3 cups finely chopped Vidalia Onions
2 cups Organic Veganaise
2 cups grated vegan Swiss cheese (Daiya brand is a good choice)
¼ teaspoon tabasco sauce
1 cup grated parmesan cheese
Paprika to taste

Preparing Dip

Preheat oven to 350 degrees. In a medium bowl mix onions, Veganaise, swiss cheese and tabasco sauce. Spread mixture into a 13 X 9 baking dish. Sprinkle with parmesan cheese and then paprika.

Bake 30 minutes until bubbly. Serve warm with veggies or your favorite cracker.

Smoothies

Vanilla Berry Breakfast Shake

This was the first shake I started making and my clients loved it. It is a great place to start eating a healthy breakfast and staying plant based. You will get 2 servings of fruits and veggies as well as omega 3's in the chia seeds and protein. You won't even know the greens are in there!

> 1 ½ cups plant milk (almond, coconut or soy)
> 1 scoop Juice Plus Vanilla Protein Powder
> 1 tablespoon chia seeds
> 1 big handful of organic baby greens (kale, spinach or romaine)
> 1 banana (optional)
> 1 cup frozen organic berries
> ½ packet organic stevia

Place all ingredients in blender and combine.

Jan's Raw Chocolate Breakfast Smoothie

This is the smoothie I have made most mornings for years. I am convinced this drink gives me my superpowers! My husband just hates hearing the Vitamix blender going every morning, but I am absolutely in love with this drink. It is raw and full of amazing antioxidants, vitamins, minerals and protein. The number of ingredients may seem daunting at first, but I keep all the dry ingredients in one cupboard and when organized, I pre-measure all the dry ingredients into individual bags with the berries in freezer and then pop in the blender. If you are not a very adventurous eater you might try my basic smoothie first and then move to this one as you get used to something a bit sweeter first.

½-1 cup organic frozen berries

1.5 cup almond milk (can use coconut, cashew or soy milk)

2 tablespoons of raw cacao powder

1-2 teaspoons acai extract powder

1 teaspoon dulse flakes

Handful of Goji Berries

2 tablespoons chia seeds or flax seeds(grind flax seeds in nut or coffee grinder for full benefit)

1 tablespoon of Maca powder

1 big handful of organic baby spinach, baby kale, or baby romaine

1 scoop raw vegan protein powder

1 packet organic stevia(or ½ tsp. Stevia powder or 4-6 drops liquid Stevia)

1 tablespoon organic coconut oil

Place all ingredients in a powerful blender and combine.

Fruit and Nut Smoothie

This shake takes only 5 minutes to prepare. Remember to soak the nuts in water the night before. It's high in protein, nice and creamy with the good fats! Makes for a good breakfast smoothie.

Servings: 1

¼ cup drained silken tofu

½ cup unsweetened almond milk

1 tablespoon organic coconut oil

2 tablespoons ground flax seeds

½ cup organic berries (strawberries, raspberries, blackberries, blueberries)

2-4 ounces filtered water

¼ cup nuts soaked overnight (such as almonds, walnuts)

Ice

Breakfast

Amish Baked Oatmeal

My stepmother, Maggie, made a version of this for me when I was visiting. It was so good I just had to play around with the ingredients to find a healthier version for my clients. The best thing about this recipe is you prepare it the night before and bake in the morning. I make it when I am having overnight guests. It's great because I pop it in the oven in the morning and my guests wake up to what smells like cookies baking! Serve with some organic berries and you'll be a hit. Keep leftovers for next day! *You can take out the flax seeds and water and replace with two organic eggs for a vegetarian version.

Serves 8

1/3 cup organic coconut oil melted

2 Tablespoons finely ground flax seeds (buy whole and grind in nut or coffee grinder)

6 Tablespoons water

3/4 cup organic coconut palm sugar

1 1/2 teaspoons baking powder

1 1/2 teaspoons vanilla

2 teaspoon cinnamon

1/4 teaspoon sea salt

1 cup unsweetened almond milk, plus 2 tablespoons

3 cups organic rolled oats

Optional: I add 1 cup raw walnuts and 1/4- 1/2 cup currants, raisins or dried cranberries. Add anything you like!

Grease 1 1/2 qt. baking dish. In medium bowl combine ground flax seeds, water, sugar, baking powder, vanilla, cinnamon and salt. Mix well, no lumps.

Whisk in melted coconut oil and both measures of milk, then add oats. Stir well and pour into greased baking dish.

Refrigerate overnight- This step is key!

Bake uncovered at 350 degrees for 35-45 minutes until set in middle. Serve hot with or without warm almond milk poured over.

Jan's Morning Rice Bowl

I just love rice in the morning. This whole grain keeps me energized until lunch, while being very digestible. You will also love that it is a leftover from the night before and requires very little work on your part and no waste. A nice break from the traditional American breakfast! A nutritional powerhouse that tastes yummy! If you are a bacon lover this will satisfy your taste for savory and salty food.

Serves 2

    1 cup leftover brown rice
    Toasted pumpkin seeds
    1/2 umeboshi plum, cut into small pieces
    Chopped fresh parsley

Place the rice in 2 cups of water in a saucepan. Bring to a boil, cover and simmer for 10 minutes. Remove from heat, pour into 2 bowls. Top by scraping small pieces of the plum on tops of each bowl of rice. Sprinkle pumpkin seeds and parsley on top.

To toast pumpkin seeds: toast shelled seeds in a dry skillet for about 5 minutes over medium heat, stirring constantly. Watch carefully so you don't burn your nuts!

Variation:

If you need a little sweetness add 4 medjool dates (chopped) in saucepan. Or any dried fruit.

Personal Sized Baked Oatmeal Muffins

This recipe was given to me by my client Randy who has Type II Diabetes. You have to love it when your clients begin to look for healthy choices for themselves! It was wonderful when he shared this gluten-free, diabetic friendly recipe with me. I adapted it from a recipe he found at SugarFreeMom.com. I make these with lots of different toppings. My daughter likes 4 chocolate chips on top, my husband dried cherries and walnuts. They are even good with no toppings at all.

Servings: 18 muffins

2 tablespoons ground flax seeds combined with 6 tablespoons water (or 2 organic eggs)

1 teaspoon vanilla extract

2 cups applesauce, unsweetened

1/2 cup or 1 ripe banana, mashed

6 packets of organic Stevia or 1 1/2 teaspoons of Stevia powder(or ½ cup raw honey if not diabetic)

5 cups, Old Fashioned rolled oats

1/4 cup chia seeds (or if using eggs ¼ cup ground flax seeds)

1 tablespoon ground cinnamon

3 teaspoons baking powder

1 teaspoon sea salt

2 1/4 cups almond or coconut milk, unsweetened

Optional toppings: raisins, walnuts, dried cranberries or chocolate chips

Preheat oven to 350 degrees.

Mix eggs, vanilla, applesauce, banana and Stevia together in a bowl. Add in oats, flax, cinnamon, baking powder, salt and mix well with wet ingredients. Finally pour in milk and combine.

Spray a 12 and 6 capacity muffin tin with cooking spray or use unbleached cupcake liners. Pour mixture evenly into muffin tin cups.

If adding toppings, place them onto the tops of muffins now. If using fresh or frozen fruit, drop it right into the batter.

Bake 30 minutes until a toothpick in center comes out clean. Cool and enjoy or freeze them in gallon freezer bags.

Jan's Cherry Granola

I created this recipe years ago and it is a crowd pleaser. I like to make it to give in mason jars for gifts. It is super yummy and a much better choice than processed cereal in a box. Buy a big jar and store it with a scoop inside.

Servings: 24

8 cups organic rolled oats
1 cup organic flax seeds
1 cup slivered raw blanched almonds
1 ½ cups raw walnuts
½ cup melted coconut oil (organic cold pressed)
1 cup organic maple syrup
1 teaspoon sea salt
2 cups dried cherries

Mix together oats, nuts and seeds, but set aside fruit. In separate bowl combine oil, syrup, salt and mix well. Add dry ingredients to wet and mix with hands or large wooden spoon. Preheat oven to 350 F. Spread mixture on baking pans to ½" deep.

Bake 14-18 minutes until top layer is browned.

Remove from oven, stir and turn, and replace in oven. Bake another 4-5 minutes, remove and stir again. Sprinkle with dried cherries.

Bake for a final 4-5 minutes and remove to large bowl. Let cool before storing.

Note: I usually use two big non-stick cookie sheets for this recipe. If yours are likely to stick, oil the pan lightly. You can use any dried fruit in this recipe. Sometimes I throw in some pumpkin seeds instead of almonds.

Soups

Pumpkin Pie Soup

This soup is all raw and gives you tons of live enzymes in a very digestible form. It has been a favorite at my cooking classes for years. It is nice and cool for the hot summer months and I flip the switch on my Vitamix blender to warm it for a first course in autumn or winter. You will need a juicer to juice the carrots before combining in a good blender (or you can buy freshly juiced carrots).

Servings: 6

      5 lb bag of organic juicing carrots, juiced
      1 ½ cup raw sweet potato, peeled and cubed
      4 medjool dates, pitted
      ½ avocado, pitted
      ½ teaspoon pumpkin pie spice

Place all of the ingredients in a high speed blender and blend until smooth. Refrigerate, enjoy now or store in an airtight container up to 24 hours.

Warming Vegetable Soup

I love this soup from fall to spring. It warms me up and is perfect for when I feel like I'm coming down with something. Feel free to substitute any veggies you have leftover in the fridge. It's impossible to mess this one up! I adapted this recipe from Alicia Silverstone's, "The Kind Diet." This has been one of my favorite cookbooks since I bought it in 2009!

Servings: 2

1 medium carrot, cut into large chunks
¼ medium daikon, cut into large chunks
¼ whole red onion, cut into large chunks
3 stalks celery, chopped
4 small broccoli florets
4 whole button mushrooms, sliced
3 whole oyster or shiitake mushrooms, sliced
½ medium leek, halved, cut into large chunks and swirled in water to dislodge grit.
1 inch piece ginger, peeled and grated
1 tablespoon Shoyu
1whole scallion, roots and all, thinly sliced on the diagonal
¼ bunch watercress, tough stems discarded
1 sheet toasted nori, torn in strips

Boil 3 cups of water in a large pot. Add the carrot and daikon. Reduce the heat to a simmer. Add the red onion, and cook for 2 to 3 minutes. Add the celery, broccoli, mushrooms, and leek. Squeeze the grated ginger juice into the broth. Then add the shoyu to the broth to taste. Simmer until the vegetables are cooked through but still slightly firm, about 5 minutes. Add the scallion, and turn off the heat.

Ladle the soup into 2 bowls. Top each serving with some watercress, and nori.

Salads and Veggies

Easy Massaged Kale

I did not grow up eating kale but now it is one of my favorite vegetables. Many years ago, this was one of the first recipes I adapted from something I saw on the internet and I'm not sure who came up with this recipe but I am grateful to whoever did. This is the recipe that made me love kale. Try it and let me know what you think!

Servings: 6

1 bunch organic kale
1/2 tsp. sea salt
¼ cup olive oil
1/3 cup currants
1/3 cup organic sunflower seeds, pine nuts, or cashew pieces, toasted
½ avocado, chopped
Splash of lemon juice

Wash kale leaves and spin or pat dry. De-stem kale by pulling from the stems. Gather the leaves, roll up, and cut into thin ribbons. Put kale in a large Ziploc bag. Add salt, zip bag and massage it into the kale with your hands for 2 minutes.

Toss currants, nuts/seeds, avocado, olive oil, lemon juice and sea salt into kale. Zip bag, allowing air in it. Shake the bag to toss. Serve and enjoy!

Superfood Kale Salad

I really like all the good things that go into this salad. I find the botija olives on Amazon. They are from Peru and unlike most olives we buy, they are raw, picked fresh and do not have chemicals added. If you don't have them you can substitute black Moroccan olives or any olive you like.

Servings: 4

1 bunch kale
1 lemon, squeezed
1 tomato, chopped
1/2 carrot, chopped
1/2 avocado
1/4 cup chopped botija olives, pitted
1/4 tsp sea salt (I like Himalayan pink)
1/4 cup dulse flakes
handful of raw cashews
handful of goji berries
handful of fresh herbs
handful of sprouts (try alfalfa, sunflower)

First, take the kale off of the stems. Place in large bowl and put salt on the leaves. Start massaging the leaves so that the salt starts to break down the leaves until they are wilted. About 2 minutes. Next, massage the leaves with lemon juice. Then, massage the leaves with the avocado until well incorporated. Taste. You might need more lemon juice or more salt. Place in serving bowl and add rest of ingredients. Enjoy!

Baby Bok Choy

Baby bok choy is chock full of calcium and very sweet. It is one of my favorite veggies and super easy to prepare. Be careful not to overcook when steaming. You want the bok choy to be a bit crunchy, but not mushy. If it is bitter you didn't cook long enough. It will continue to cook a bit even after you turn off the heat. The ume plum vinegar is a wonderful fermented vinegar and can be found at most health food stores. Gomashio is a delicious condiment you can buy already made or you can make your own, it is really easy. Gomasio is full of vitamins and minerals and aids digestion.

Servings: 2

2 whole heads of baby bok choy
1 1/2 teaspoons of extra-virgin olive oil
1 1/2 teaspoons umeboshi plum vinegar
1 teaspoon Gomashio (optional)

Place a steamer basket in bottom of a large pot or in a steamer pot, add an inch or two of water. Bring water to a boil, and add baby bok choy. Steam for 1-2 minutes until just beginning to wilt. Transfer to serving dish.

Whisk vinegar and oil together in a small bowl, and drizzle over steamed bok choy. Sprinkle with gomasio.

Sweet Potatoes with Lime and Cilantro

Ever since I learned that white potatoes were part of the white menace, I started eating sweet potatoes instead. They satisfy my craving for something sweet and I like this recipe as a change from the traditional ways of preparing sweet potatoes, e.g.,brown sugar, marshmallows, etc. I especially like anything with lime and cilantro! The perfect pairing that is so fresh tasting.

Servings: 4

4 sweet potatoes

1/2 bunch fresh cilantro

2-3 limes

Olive oil, salt (optional)

Wash sweet potatoes, poke with a knife or fork, and bake them whole, in their skins, at 375 degrees until tender, about 45 minutes.

Wash and chop cilantro leaves.

When sweet potatoes are done, slit open the skin and place on serving plate. Season with salt, drizzle with a bit of oil, then squeeze fresh lime juice all over, and cover with cilantro leaves.

Entrées

Baked Falafel Lettuce Wraps with Lemon Tahini Sauce

These little bites are a real crowd pleaser and perfect because I can make them ahead, freeze in servings, and pull out on busy days as needed. I like that they are baked and not fried. Warm them up, wrap in lettuce with some tomatoes, shredded carrots, pickle, and my lemon tahini sauce and you have an easy meal.

Servings: 20 bite-sized falafel

3 cloves garlic, peeled
1/2 cup onion
1/3 cup fresh cilantro, packed
1/3 cup fresh parsley, packed
1 (15 oz) can garbanzo beans, drained and rinsed
1 tablespoon coconut oil, organic, expeller pressed
2 tablespoons ground flaxseed
1/2 cup spelt or gluten-free bread crumbs
1/2 teaspoon ground cumin
1/2 teaspoon sea salt

Preheat oven to 400 degrees. Line baking sheet with parchment paper. Wrap onion in cheese cloth and squeeze out as much moisture as you can. Set aside.

In food processor, pulse garlic to finely chop. Add onion, cilantro, parsley, and process until fine. Add garbanzos and coconut oil and process until mixture holds together in a course dough.

Transfer to a large bowl, add ground flaxseed, 1/4 cup of the bread crumbs, cumin and sea salt. Mix with your hands to combine.

Shape into small patties about 1-2 tablespoons in size. Brush a small amount of water on each patty and roll in remaining bread crumbs.

Bake until golden, about 25-30 minutes, turning halfway through cooking time.

Serve with lemon tahini sauce, shredded carrots, pickle and sliced tomatoes on Bibb or Romaine lettuce leaves.

Lemon Tahini Sauce (Makes about 1 cup)

1/2 cup sesame tahini

3 large garlic cloves

5 tablespoons fresh squeezed lemon juice

2-6 tablespoons water

3/4 teaspoon sea salt

In food processor, place tahini, garlic, 4 tablespoons of the lemon juice and 2 tablespoons of water. Blend well, scraping sides as needed and adding additional water and/or lemon juice to create a thick sauce that still has a pourable consistency. Add the salt and stir.

Make ahead and refrigerate up to one week. Double up the recipe and use as topping for other meals.

Red Quinoa

This is a great main course dish, economical, and super simple for a quick weekday meal. Steam some broccoli, toss a green salad and you've got a nutritional powerhouse meal! Quinoa is a complete protein, so think of it as the "meat" of the meal. I like red quinoa as I find it has a nuttier texture than the white version.

Servings: 6

1 cup red quinoa

1 1/2 cups water

Pinch of sea salt

2 tablespoons extra virgin olive oil

1 small yellow onion, chopped

1/2 cup currants

3 dashes ume plum vinegar

Rinse quinoa and drain. Place quinoa in pot with water, salt and bring to a boil. Cover, reduce to simmer and cook until water is absorbed (about 15 minutes). Don't overcook. Remove from heat, cool slightly, then fluff with fork.

In large skillet, heat 1 tablespoon olive oil over medium heat until shimmering. Add the onion and sauté until soft (about 3 minutes). Add currants and sauté another 3 minutes. Fold in the cooked quinoa to combine ingredients. Add remaining tablespoon of olive oil and 3 dashes of plum vinegar and serve.

Garlic Tofu With Orange Marmalade

I like a crispy tofu that tastes garlicky and this marmalade dip makes this main course a bit sweet with no added sugar. If you have never liked tofu before, give this recipe a try. I cook this in my iron skillet as it comes out a bit crispier. This also makes a great appetizer to serve with the dipping sauce. Arrange on a narrow rectangle serving dish with some chopsticks for dipping.This recipe was adapted from Angela Liddon's, *The Oh She Glows Cookbook*.

Servings: 4

1 block extra-firm tofu (organic and sprouted if possible)

1 ½ teaspoons garlic powder

¼ teaspoon sea salt

¼ teaspoon fresh ground black pepper

1 tablespoon melted coconut oil

4 tablespoons of St. Dalfour Marmalade 100% fruit preserves (or other whole fruit brand)

Tofu

Drain tofu, wrap in paper towels, and then in a kitchen towel and set something heavy on it for 25-30 minutes to absorb the water or use a tofu press. Slice tofu into 9 or 10 rectangles and then cut each rectangle into 6 squares.

Preheat skillet over medium-high heat.

In a medium size bowl, combine tofu, garlic powder, salt, and pepper. Toss until coated.

Add coconut oil to skillet and spread to edges of pan. Add tofu squares to pan in a single layer. Cook 3-5 minutes on each side until they are golden.

Dipping Sauce

Place marmalade in small saucepan with 3 tablespoons of water over medium heat. Stir and warm through, do not boil. Divide among 4 small dipping bowls.

Almond Flaxseed Burger

These burgers can be made in about 10 minutes. Serve raw or cooked. I prefer them raw because they retain all of their enzyme content when raw. If you choose to serve them cooked, say, in winter months, lightly spray with coconut oil and bake at 300 degrees for 35 minutes. I like them with the pineapple salsa on the next page.

Servings: 2

2 cloves garlic
1 cup almonds
1/2 cup ground flaxseed
2 tablespoons balsamic vinegar
2 tablespoons coconut oil
Pinch of sea salt

Place all ingredients into a food processor. Process until well blended. Form into 2 patties.

Pineapple Salsa

This salsa is a nice topping for the raw burger but can also be used to top chicken or tofu. Keep refrigerated for up to 1 week.

Servings: 12

1/2 jalapeño, chopped
2 cups cubed pineapple
1/2 cup chopped red bell pepper
1/4 cup diced Spanish onion
1 tablespoon chopped cilantro
1 tablespoon fresh lime juice
1 tablespoon hemp oil
1 teaspoon lime zest

Process in food processor until blended but still chunky.

Afterword

I wrote this book because I can't help but look around and see how many people are suffering. They are struggling with weight, lethargy, depression and the dread of growing older. I feel compassion for these people in their struggles, confusion, stress and lack of health and with the financial burden this places on them. My hope is that some of the ideas presented here will make even a small difference in their lives. For those of you who are already healthy lifestyle lovers, I hope this book serves as a bit of inspiration to keep you moving on the continuum towards health.

I am blessed to coach people every day who are working hard to become better versions of themselves. It's not easy to undo years of bad habits in a society that has it all wrong with regard to eating and how we move. I am humbled by the trust my clients place in me to guide them.

Interested in having Jan Rodenfels speak at your next event?

Email for a list of topics at jan@janyourcoach.com

Check out her website at www.janyourcoach.com

Follow JanYourCoach on Instagram

Acknowledgments

I would like to thank all of those who supported me in the writing of this book when all I am really capable of is helping people get well. This has been quite a journey with my first book and there are many people to thank for supporting me.

To my husband, Charlie, who supports me in all my endeavors, including this book. I can't begin to tell you how much I love and appreciate your patience with all my ideas, projects and sometimes, my too full plate. You have always let me go and do what I want and that's why I will always come back to you. You are the love of my life. Thank you for supporting whatever new adventure I embark on. For all the meals you prepared, dishes you washed and tears you wiped away, it is because of you that I could complete this project. To my daughters, Courtney and Alexandra, you are truly the joys of my life. You are both beautiful young women with beautiful hearts. It's for you and all people, both young and old, that I write for a healthier life and planet.

I would like to acknowledge my parents for their love and devotion; and for teaching me important life lessons as well as a good work ethic. A big thanks to my sisters, Denise, Brenda and Krista for helping to make me who I am. I am blessed to have all of you in my life!

My friends were my biggest cheerleaders throughout this project. Their words of encouragement kept me on task and believing I could do this project. They loved me and were patient even when I disappeared into my cave to write and they know who they are.

Many thanks to my team who helped me with this book. Susan Edison, my cover designer who is enormously talented and who I knew I could trust with this project. Kyle Widder of KDWPhoto who made me look good even without retouching! Susan Fortner, publicist extraordinaire. Stephanie Schlie, my talented editor. My intern, Emily Bichsel, whose help allowed me the time to begin this book.

I'm grateful for the contributions from Howard Lyman, Nick Baird, Jack and Suzi Hanna. And I can't leave out Lindsay Smith and Joshua Rosenthal; if it weren't for them this book would still be in my head.

Recommended Reading

Books

The Blood Sugar Solution, Mark Hyman, M.D.

The China Study, T. Colin Campbell, Ph.D., Thomas M. Campbell, II

Diet for a Poisoned Planet, David Steinman

Fast Food Nation, Eric Schlosser

Healing With Whole Foods, Paul Pitchford

Mad Cowboy, Howard F. Lyman with Glen Merzer

No More Bull, Howard F. Lyman with Glen Merzer

Slaughterhouse, Gail A. Eisnitz

The Third Plate, Dan Barber

Thrive, Brendan Brazier

The Way We Eat, Peter Singer and Jim Mason

Spiritual/ Self-Help Books

The Alchemist, Paulo Coelho

The Bible

Creating True Prosperity, Shakti Gawain

Everything Belongs, Richard Rohr

Falling Upward, Richard Rohr

Frederick, Frederick Ndabaramiye and Amy Parker

Learned Optimism, Martin E. P. Seligman, Ph.D.

Reinventing the Body, Resurrecting the Soul, Deepak Chopra

The Shack, William P. Young

Tuesdays With Morrie, Mitch Albom

DVDs/Documentaries

Food, Inc.

Forks Over Knives

Hungry For Change

Mad Cowboy

Veducated

Cookbooks

Clean Food, Terry Walters

Deliciously Ella, Ella Woodward

Eat Clean Live Well, Terry Walters

The Kind Diet, Alicia Silverstone

The Oh She Glows Cookbook, Angela Liddon

Vegan Delights, Jeanne Marie Martin

NOTES

10 Simple Tips to Balance Blood Sugar | Reboot With Joe. (2014, October 24). Retrieved from http://www.rebootwithjoe.com/10-simple-tips-to-balance-blood-sugar/

15 Ways Puppies Improve Your Life. (n.d.). Retrieved from http://www.shape.com/lifestyle/mind-and-body/top-15-ways-puppies-improve-your-health

18 Surprising Dairy-Free Sources of Calcium. (n.d.). Retrieved from http://greatist.com/health/18-surprising-dairy-free-sources-calcium

54 Million Americans Affected by Osteoporosis and Low Bone Mass. (2014, June 2). Retrieved from http://nof.org/news/2948

Added Sugars. (n.d.). Retrieved from http://www.heart.org/HEARTORG/HealthyLiving/HealthyEating/Nutrition/Added-Sugars_UCM_305858_Article.jsp#.Vtywi8d-GFI

Albom, M. (1997). *Tuesdays with Morrie: An old man, a young man, and life's greatest lesson.* New York: Doubleday.

Britt, R. R. (2006, April 03). Churchgoers Live Longer. Retrieved from http://www.livescience.com/4017-churchgoers-live-longer.html

Cache Cab: Taxi Drivers' Brains Grow to Navigate London's Streets. (n.d.). Retrieved from http://www.scientificamerican.com/article/london-taxi-memory/

Campbell, T. C., & Campbell, T. M. (2005). *The China study: The most comprehensive study of nutrition ever conducted and the startling implications for diet, weight loss and long-term health.* Dallas, TX: BenBella Books.

Casey, J. (n.d.). Do you know how much sugar you're eating? Retrieved from http://www.medicinenet.com/script/main/art.asp?articlekey=56589

Chilkov, D. N. (n.d.). Avocados: A Super Cancer Fighting Food. Retrieved from http://www.huffingtonpost.com/nalini-chilkov/avocados-a-super-cancer-f_b_632985.html

Colorectal Cancer. (n.d.). Retrieved from http://www.aicr.org/learn-more-about-cancer/colorectal-cancer/

Coso, D. (2010). Active Passive Recovery between Long Duration (40 to 120 s) Sprints. Retrieved from http://www.nataswim.info/athletic/articles/481-active-passive-recovery-long-duration.html

European Journal of Aging. Retrieved from http://www.springer.com/alert/
urltracking.do?id=L3dd0ad7Md461a0Sb0c17d1

Exercise or Physical Activity. (2016, February 10). Retrieved from http://www.cdc.gov/
nchs/fastats/exercise.htm

The Facts About RisingHealth Care Costs. (n.d.). Retrieved from http://www.aetna.
com/health-reform-connection/aetnas-vision/facts-about-costs.html

Falls and Injury Statistics for Seniors and Elderly. (n.d.). Retrieved from http://www.
learnnottofall.com/content/fall-facts/how-often.jsp

Fitness articles. (n.d.). Retrieved from http://www.womenfitness.net/shed_pounds.
htm

Food, Nutrition, Physical Activity, and the prevention of Cancer. (n.d.). Retrieved
from http://www.aicr.org/research/research_science_expert_report.html

Fox, M. (n.d.). Dairy, Supplements Do Little For Bones, Study Finds. Retrieved from
http://www.nbcnews.com/health/diet-fitness/calcium-supplements-or-dairy-
doesnt-strengthen-bones-study-finds-n435726

Goodman, B. (n.d.). Study Ties Too Much Sitting to Risks for Certain Cancers.
Retrieved from http://consumer.healthday.com/mental-health-information-25/
behavior-health-news-56/study-ties-too-much-sitting-to-risks-for-certain-
cancers-688886.html

Gregoire, C. (2014, February 25). 7 Cultures That Celebrate Aging And Respect
Their Elders. Retrieved February 18, 2016, from http://www.huffingtonpost.
com/2014/02/25/what-other-cultures-can-teach_n_4834228.html

Hatherill, J. R. (1998). *Eat to beat cancer*. Los Angeles, CA, CA: Renaissance Books.

HealthDay, W. N. (n.d.). Can Selenium Lower Risk of Advanced Prostate
Cancer? – WebMD. Retrieved from http://www.webmd.com/prostate-cancer/
news/20130409/can-selenium-lower-risk-of-advanced-prostate-cancer

High milk diet 'may not cut risk of bone fractures' - BBC News. (n.d.). Retrieved from
http://www.bbc.com/news/health-29805374

How Bread with Refined White Flour Affects Your Health. (n.d.). Retrieved from
http://articles.mercola.com/sites/articles/archive/2011/06/30/we-have-known-
bread-has-been-bad-for-your-health-for-over-a-century.aspx

Hyman, M. (2012). *The blood sugar solution: The ultrahealthy program for losing weight,
preventing disease, and feeling great now!* New York, NY: Little, Brown and.

Hyman, M. M. (n.d.). Magnesium: The Most Powerful Relaxation Mineral Available.
Retrieved from http://www.huffingtonpost.com/dr-mark-hyman/magnesium-
the-most-powerf_b_425499.html

Importance of Healthy Breakfast: Why Skipping Is Harmful. (n.d.). Retrieved from http://www.webmd.com/food-recipes/most-important-meal

Introduction. (2015, December). Retrieved March 6, 2016, from http://health.gov/dietaryguidelines/2015/guidelines/introduction/a-roadmap-to-the-2015-2020-edition-of-the-dietary-guidelines-for-americans/

Kaur, C., & Kapoor, H. C. (2001). Antioxidants in fruits and vegetables-the millennium's health. *International Journal of Food Science and Technology*, 703-725.

Klein, S., & Morin, K. (n.d.). 6 Foods That Will Protect You From The Sun. Retrieved from http://www.huffingtonpost.com/2013/07/10/sun-protection-foods_n_3568707.html

Kubota, Y., Iso, H., & Sawoda, N. (n.d.). Research_science_expert_report | American Institute for Cancer Research (AICR). Retrieved from http://www.aicr.org/research/research_science_expert_report.html

LeWine, H., M.D. (2014, April 04). Benefits of vitamin D supplements still debated - Harvard Health Blog. Retrieved from http://www.health.harvard.edu/blog/benefits-vitamin-d-supplements-still-debated-201404047106

Liddon, A. (2015). *Oh She Glows*. Penguin Books.

Lindeberg, S., Nilsson-ehle, P., & Vessby, B. (n.d.). Lipoprotein composition and serum cholesterol ester fatty acids in nonwesternized Melanesians. Retrieved from https://www.researchgate.net/publication/14370795_Lipoprotein_composition_and_serum_cholesterol_ester_fatty_acids_in_nonwesternized_Melanesians

Lindeberg, S., Nilsson-Elle, P., Terént, A., Vessby, B., & Scherstén, B. (n.d.). TheKitavaStudy. Retrieved from http://www.staffanlindeberg.com/TheKitavaStudy.html

Linden, B. (2011). Fruit and vegetable intake and coronary heart disease Crowe F, Roddam AW, Key T et al for the EPIC Heart Study Investigators (2011) Fruit and vegetable intake and mortality from ischaemic heart disease: Results from the European Prospective Investigation into Cancer and Nutrition (EPIC)-Heart study . Eur Heart J 10.1093/eurheartj/ehq465 (online ahead of print). *Br J Cardiac Nursing British Journal of Cardiac Nursing*, 6(4), 202-202. doi:10.12968/bjca.2011.6.4.202

Lyman, H. F., & Merzer, G. (1998). *Mad cowboy.: Plain truth from the cattle rancher who won't eat meat*. New York, NY: Scribner.

MacGill, M. (n.d.). Oxytocin-what it is & what does it do? Retrieved from http://www.medicalnewstoday.com/articles/275795.php

Marcela, Dr. (n.d.). Magnesium: The Missing Link to Better Health. Retrieved from http://articles.mercola.com/sites/articles/archive/2013/12/08/magnesium-health-benefits.aspx

Mcguffin, L. E., Price, R. K., Mccaffrey, T. A., Hall, G., Lobo, A., Wallace, J. M., & Livingstone, M. B. (2014). Parent and child perspectives on family out-of-home eating: A qualitative analysis. *Public Health Nutr. Public Health Nutrition,* 18(01), 100-111. doi:10.1017/s1368980014001384

Mendes, E. (2014). Adults Take In 200 More Calories Per Day When They Eat Out. Retrieved from http://www.cancer.org/research/acsresearchupdates/cancerprevention/adults-take-in-about-200-extra-calories-per-day-when-they-eat-out

Ndabaramiye, F., & Parker, A. (2014). *Frederick: A story of boundless hope.* Nashville, TN: W. Publishing Group.

Negative Effects of "Skipping Breakfast" (n.d.). Retrieved from http://www.powershow.com/view/45b23a-ZTJiY/Negative_Effects_of_Skipping_Breakfast_powerpoint_ppt_presentation

Physical Actvity Epidemiology 2E: Individual barriers to physical activity influence behavior. (n.d.). Retrieved from http://www.humankinetics.com/excerpts/excerpts/individual-barriers-to-physical-activity-influence-behavior-

Pitchford, P. (2002). *Healing With Whole Foods* (3rd ed.). Berkeley, CA: North Atlantic Books.

Pollan, M. (2008). *In defense of food: An eater's manifesto.* New York, NY: Penguin Press.

Providing Social Support May Be More Beneficial Than Receiving It. (n.d.). Retrieved from http://www.psychologicalscience.org/pdf/14_4Brown.cfm

Schmid, D., & Leitzmann, M. F. (2014). Television Viewing and Time Spent Sedentary in Relation to Cancer Risk: A Meta-analysis. *JNCI Journal of the National Cancer Institute,* 106(7). doi:10.1093/jnci/dju098

Schmidt, L. (n.d.). New USDA Dietary Guidelines Validated by UCSF Sugar Research. Retrieved from https://www.ucsf.edu/news/2016/01/401326/new-usda-dietary-guidelines-validated-ucsf-sugar-research

Silverstone, A., & Pearson, V. (2009). *The kind diet: A simple guide to feeling great, losing weight, and saving the planet.* Emmaus, PA: Rodale.

Skipping breakfast may increase coronary heart disease risk. (2013, July 23). Retrieved from http://www.hsph.harvard.edu/news/features/skipping-breakfast-may-increase-coronary-heart-disease-risk/

Skipping breakfast may increase coronary heart disease risk. (2013, July 23). Retrieved from http://www.hsph.harvard.edu/news/features/skipping-breakfast-may-increase-coronary-heart-disease-risk/

Stenson, J. (2005, July 12). Exercise may make you a better worker. Retrieved from http://www.nbcnews.com/id/8160459/ns/health-fitness/t/exercise-may-make-you-better-worker/#.Vt2IgMd-GFJ

Stress in America: Our Health at Risk. (n.d.). *PsycEXTRA Dataset.* doi:10.1037/e506172012-001

Times, T. A. (n.d.). Sitting Is the New Smoking: Ways a Sedentary Lifestyle Is Killing You. Retrieved from http://www.huffingtonpost.com/the-active-times/sitting-is-the-new-smokin_b_5890006.html

Trichopoulou, A. (2005). Modified Mediterranean diet and survival: Author's reply. Bmj, 330(7503), 1329-1330. doi:10.1136/bmj.330.7503.1329-b

An Unhealthy America: The Economic Burden of Chronic Disease -- Charting a New Course to Save Lives and Increase Productivity and Economic Growth. (n.d.). Retrieved from http://www.milkeninstitute.org/publications/view/321

Walnuts | The New Breast Cancer Fighting Food - Integrative Cancer Answers. (2012, August 25). Retrieved from http://www.integrativecanceranswers.com/walnuts-the-new-breast-cancer-fighting-food/

Warming Up to Winter Exercise. (n.d.). Retrieved from http://www.sparkpeople.com/resource/pregnancy_articles.asp?ID=998

Watkins, E. (2015, August 23). Acidifying Foods & Inflammation. Retrieved March 6, 2016, from http://www.livestrong.com/article/548288-acidifying-foods-inflammation/

Weil, A., Dr. (n.d.). Need a News Fast? Retrieved from http://www.drweil.com/drw/u/QAA401018/Need-a-News-Fast.html

What Sugar Does to Your Body. (n.d.). Retrieved from http://www.womenshealthmag.com/health/how-sugar-affects-the-body

Whitelocks, S. (n.d.). Why fish is good for your brain: Study suggests it can make Alzheimer's far less likely. Retrieved from http://www.dailymail.co.uk/health/article-2067597/Why-fish-oil-good-brain-Study-finds-boosts-memory-15-cent.html

Why is it important to eat fruit? (2015, March 8). Retrieved February 18, 2016, from http://www.choosemyplate.gov/food-groups/fruits-why.html

Your body language shapes who you are. (n.d.). Retrieved from http://www.ted.com/talks/amy_cuddy_your_body_language_shapes_who_you_are